Z₂
med

12/26

*Breastfeeding and HIV/AIDS*

# Breastfeeding and HIV/AIDS

## The Research, the Politics, the Women's Responses

*by* EDITH WHITE

McFarland & Company, Inc., Publishers
*Jefferson, North Carolina, and London*

British Library Cataloguing-in-Publication data are available

Library of Congress Cataloguing-in-Publication Data

White, Edith, 1943–
  Breastfeeding and HIV/AIDS : the research, the politics, the
women's responses / by Edith White.
      p.   cm.
    Includes bibliographical references and index.
    ISBN 0-7864-0694-1 (sewn softcover : 50# alkaline paper) ∞
    1. AIDS (Disease) in infants — Etiology.   2. Breast feeding —
Health aspects.   3. AIDS (Disease) in women.   4. AIDS
(Disease) — Transmission.   5. AIDS (Disease) in women —
Political aspects.   I. Title.
RJ387.A25W43   1999
618.82'9792071— dc21                                        99-13982
                                                                        CIP

Manufactured in the United States of America

*McFarland & Company, Inc., Publishers
  Box 611, Jefferson, North Carolina 28640*

To my daughter
Amy Tibbetts

With a thank you for editing
and with fond memories of
our two and a half years of breastfeeding

# Contents

# Introduction

In this book I focus on breastfeeding as it relates to HIV/AIDS, because this issue has been largely overlooked. Yet HIV transmission through breastfeeding involves the lives of millions of babies.

I bring to the topic both passion and relative expertise, having worked full-time in the field of breastfeeding education since 1974, co-authored *The Breastfeeding Handbook: A Practical Reference for Physicians, Nurses and Other Health Professionals* (1980, 1989) and written breastfeeding pamphlets that have sold by the hundreds of thousands. I participated in the U.S. Surgeon General's Workshop on Breastfeeding and Human Lactation, 1984. In 1985, I was one of a small group of women who pioneered the field of lactation consulting, and was "grandmothered" in as one of the original International Board Certified Lactation Consultants (IBCLC). I was one of three members of the External Review Board for "Baby Friendly USA," which is part of UNICEF's global breastfeeding initiative. I have been deeply involved with breastfeeding every day for more than twenty years.

Like most U.S. breastfeeding advocates, I learned in the mid–1980s that breastfeeding could transmit the AIDS virus. But also like most breastfeeding advocates, I thought that breastfeeding played a small part in mother-to-child HIV transmission until I read the original research. Over the years, I read more and more research, and what I learned horrified me. Babies who were breast-fed long-term by HIV-infected mothers stood a very significant risk of becoming HIV-infected, *not* a minor risk as I had been led to believe.

I had reviewed hundreds of articles about HIV in infants and was deeply troubled by what I'd read by the time I left for Thailand in November 1996.

1

I had been chosen by UNICEF as one of the two people to represent the United States at an international breastfeeding colloquium in Bangkok. It was the first training conference about breastfeeding ever held and was sponsored by UNICEF, the World Health Organization and the World Alliance for Breastfeeding Action (WABA). During the colloquium, we didn't mention HIV, even when we talked about the breastfeeding practices of Africans. One estimate was that AIDS would triple child mortality rates in Zambia, but we seemed to be pretending we'd never heard of AIDS. I sat there wondering how meaningful our discussions really were. The topic of AIDS came up only once, when a physician asked how HIV-positive women in Thailand were feeding their babies. A UNICEF representative said the Thai government was supplying free formula, but that the government was wrong to allow the mothers to use baby bottles to feed the formula. Our Thai obstetrician-hostess was told, in no uncertain terms, that she should make HIV-positive mothers cup-feed formula, rather than bottle-feed formula, since baby bottles can become dirty and contaminated. And, someone added, other (HIV-negative) mothers who saw baby bottles might want them too, possibly hurting breastfeeding promotion efforts. If people had been walking outside in the hall during the heated discussion, they might have heard shouts of "Charcoal! Charcoal!" Mothers in Thailand use charcoal to heat water to mix with formula and sterilize baby bottles. Doing this, to the agitation of a representative of UNICEF, wastes charcoal.

A Breastfeeding Global Forum was held the second week in Bangkok. I was a speaker and discussed the "Report Card on the State of Breastfeeding in the United States," which I had written. During the weeklong conference, only twenty minutes were spent on breastfeeding and AIDS. The keynote speaker, a pediatrician from Uganda who had been asked to fill in at the last minute, gave a good overview of the data. He received, however, a very chilly reaction and dirty looks from the audience of breastfeeding advocates, who apparently had hoped to hear that HIV transmission via breastfeeding was not a major problem. He — who had toiled endlessly in the cause of breastfeeding in Africa — was glared at. He was neither thanked nor applauded, although all the other presenters were. It seemed like a classic case of kill the messenger.

After the talk, in the hallway, one of the delegates from Zimbabwe told me that women in her country were already abandoning breastfeeding. They hadn't been tested for HIV, but they were avoiding breastfeeding because of the rumors that breastmilk transmitted the AIDS virus. The woman whispered to me that women's groups in Zimbabwe were accusing breastfeeding advocates of "killing babies" by telling them to breastfeed. There is graffiti on the walls saying, "UNICEF kills babies."

The experience in Bangkok was a turning point for me. I came back to the United States very unsettled. What I heard in my home nation disturbed me further. An HIV-positive woman told our local county health meeting on

Cape Cod about her HIV-positive friend who breastfed against doctor's orders because she did not believe that breastfeeding can transmit HIV. Now she has to live with guilt; she thinks her infected child contracted the virus from breastmilk.

I spent the next year teaching weeklong breastfeeding training programs and found that U.S. breastfeeding advocates were not familiar with the research. A few confessed to me that they had been telling HIV-positive women to go ahead and breastfeed. Later I learned that the HIV Law Project had initiated a class action lawsuit against New York State on behalf of HIV-positive women who were breastfeeding for weeks before they were informed that they were HIV-positive.

A woman who works with United Nations programs offered to arrange a meeting for me with some wives of African ambassadors. The meeting never took place. The African women said that they were afraid UNICEF, which controlled considerable funding in their countries, might find out that they had done the unacceptable in talking about HIV and breastfeeding.

I write this book because I believe that having more open discussion about breastfeeding and HIV is necessary. While transmission through breastfeeding is tragic, it is preventable. The world community can not only do more to keep women from becoming HIV-infected; it can also do a better job in helping HIV-infected women to feed their babies safely. Clearly it is a terrible status quo to have uninfected women in Africa abandon breastfeeding while some HIV-positive women in countries such as the United States breastfeed.

Questions need answers, so I hope to stimulate discussion on these: Are babies of HIV-infected mothers in resource-poor countries better off with or without breastfeeding? What does the research say? What do the mothers say? Why do some women breastfeed even though they know that their milk can infect their babies? Why are some uninfected mothers in resource-poor countries risking their babies' lives by bottle-feeding them? Who should decide how women feed their babies? If medical personnel start to recommend formula for babies of HIV-positive mothers, will other mothers take this as a general endorsement of formula-feeding? How badly is HIV going to undermine breastfeeding efforts? And what can the world community do to minimize the consequences?

# PART ONE:

# AIDS Research

CHAPTER ONE

———————

# HIV Transmission
# Rates Among Breast
# Versus Bottle-Fed Babies

Breastfeeding offers tremendous benefits for mothers and babies. But breast milk, like blood or semen, is a body fluid that can transmit the human immunodeficiency virus (HIV). This book will present the evidence available through mid–1998. Women who are HIV-positive do not always transmit the virus to their babies during pregnancy, during childbirth, or through breastfeeding. But breastfeeding increases the chances of infection significantly. When HIV-positive women have babies and bottle-feed them, they transmit the virus in approximately 15–25 percent of the cases. These women transmit the virus during their pregnancy (*in utero*) or, more often, during labor and delivery (*intrapartum*). When they are treated with drugs such as AZT, HIV-positive women transmit the virus in only 2–8 percent of the cases, if they avoid breastfeeding. But when HIV-positive women have babies and breastfeed them, they transmit the virus in approximately 25–45 percent of the cases.

In 1985, the United States Centers for Disease Control and Prevention (CDC) was the first agency to advise HIV-infected women not to breastfeed, and other industrialized countries did the same. Some intermediate countries such as Brazil and Thailand also recommended that HIV-positive women avoid breastfeeding. The recommendations from Brazil were unequivocal: "Every human being, without distinction, has the right to a standard of living capable of ensuring adequate health. Consequently, it is utterly impracticable to

accept the possibility that HIV-infected mothers breastfeed their babies"
(Health Ministry 1995).

## UNAIDS: The Global AIDS Program

Previously, the World Health Organization (WHO) had advised *all* women
in developing countries to breastfeed, even if they were HIV-infected (WHO
1987, World Health Organization Global Programme 1992). But universal
breastfeeding for all HIV-infected women has not been the policy since 1996
(UNAIDS 1996), when the policy changed to informed choice.

The name UNAIDS stands for the Joint United Nations Program on
HIV/AIDS. It is a global effort program cosponsored with the World Health
Organization, UNICEF, World Bank, and other United Nations (UN) agencies.
UNAIDS replaced the WHO's Global Program on AIDS, January 1, 1996. Statements
now come from UNAIDS, but in conjunction with the WHO, UNICEF and other
United Nations agencies.

In 1996, UNAIDS, with UNICEF and the WHO, issued the interim recommendation that HIV-positive women, including those in resource-poor countries, be given information and be allowed to make their own decision about
how they feed their babies. The World Health Organization published this
statement in September 1996. In May 1997 it became a Policy Statement:

> Counseling for women who are aware of their HIV status should include
> the best available information on the benefits of breast-feeding, on the
> risk of HIV transmission through breast-feeding, and the risks and pos-
> sible advantages associated with other methods of infant feeding.

Then each woman can decide for herself. The statement also recommended
that, as a general rule in all populations, breastfeeding should continue to be
protected, promoted and supported. In November 1997 UNAIDS (1997b) issued
an additional statement, entitled "Breastfeeding and HIV/AIDS," reporting that
breastfeeding more than doubled the risk of mother-to-child HIV transmission:

> Recent data from developing countries indicates that up to one half
> of mother-to-child HIV transmission is due to breastfeeding. One
> South African study, for example, found that mother-to-child trans-
> mission of HIV infection was 17% for babies who were fed with infant
> formula (who are likely to have contracted HIV during pregnancy or
> at birth) and 38% for breast-fed babies (21% of whom are likely to
> have contracted the virus from breastmilk).

In December 1997, UNAIDS noted that it had grossly underestimated
HIV/AIDS, conceding that HIV infection was "far more common in the world

than previously thought" (UNAIDS 1997d). There are over 30 million people living with HIV infection: one in every 100 adults (aged 15–49 years) world-wide. But of the 30 million, 27 million do not know that they are infected. Of the 2.3 million people who died of AIDS in 1997, 46 percent were women and 460,000 were children.

The CDC (1998) noted that UNAIDS' estimates on mother-to-child trans-mission may be too conservative. While UNAIDS reported that 590,000 chil-dren were HIV-infected by their mothers in 1997, CDC noted that the total is higher if transmission through breastmilk is taken into account. The CDC esti-mated that an additional 273,000 to 410,000 children would be HIV-infected through breastmilk in 1998.

All HIV-positive women, UNAIDS recommended, should be advised of the risk of transmitting the virus to their children, and if they choose not to breastfeed, they should be assisted in their choice not to do so. This includes helping HIV-positive women in resource-poor countries to make safe use of alternatives to breastfeeding.

The countries where the HIV/AIDS pandemic is worst are the same coun-tries where bottle-feeding is least safe and least affordable. The highest rates of HIV/AIDS continue to be in sub–Saharan Africa, that is, Africa south of the Sahara Desert. Rates of infection are now expanding rapidly in Asia. India today has more cases of HIV, though not a correspondingly higher rate of infection, than any other single country. Ninety-seven percent of all HIV-infected women live in Africa, Asia and Latin America, where breastfeeding is routine.

Rates of HIV infection are particularly high among *women* in sub–Saharan Africa. One report from UNAIDS was that there were already six HIV-infected women for every five infected men in the arid region (UNAIDS 1997a). In much of sub–Saharan Africa, 15–25 percent of pregnant women are HIV-infected, and in some urban areas the figure is as high as 40 percent (UNAIDS 1997d). One prenatal clinic in Zimbabwe reported that seven out of ten pregnant women were HIV-infected.

In a growing number of countries, it is AIDS— not lack of breastfeeding — that is the leading cause of child deaths (UNAIDS 1998). One estimate is that the peak of the AIDS epidemic will come in the year 2010. At that time, AIDS will cause 41 percent of all infant deaths in Kenya, 58 percent in Zimbabwe, and 61 percent in Botswana (Piot 1997).

Of the 16,000 new HIV infections discovered each day, 40 percent occur in women of childbearing age (Luzuriaga 1998). The greatest number of new infections among women affects those between the ages of 15 and 24 years, reflecting partly the male preference for younger sexual partners. Thus women are becoming HIV-infected just before or during their childbearing years, and the issue of breastfeeding, or not breastfeeding, by these women involves the lives of literally millions of babies.

## To Protect Babies, Protect Women

The best way to protect babies from becoming HIV-infected is to protect women from becoming HIV-infected. For every case of mother-to-child transmission, there is an HIV-infected woman. Non-infected children who are orphaned by the death of their parents still fare badly.

Many women become HIV-infected through sex with their husband or boyfriend. Many infected women had only one sexual partner in the year of infection. Male-to-female transmission via semen is more efficient than female-to-male transmission via cervicovaginal secretions. Women in most of the world are also more vulnerable because they often have little or no control over whether to have sexual intercourse, or whether a condom will be used. Nor do women usually have control over the extracurricular sexual activities of their male partners or the economic freedom to leave men on whom they and their children are dependent.

The development of an effective vaccine, which might protect women, and men and children, is still some time away and is expected to provide a much lower level of defense than immunizations for simpler microbes such as polio or smallpox. Dr. Arthur Ammann, president of the American Foundation for AIDS Research, noted, "Perhaps the most we can expect is 50% protection" (Ammann 1997). Vaccines for other *viral* diseases do not block infection, but rather protect against the development of disease after infection occurs. The hope is that an HIV/AIDS vaccine will inhibit the rampant viral multiplication that occurs after infection.

There is also no guarantee that vaccines will be affordable for people in the countries most affected. Dutch virologist Jaap Goudsmit noted in his 1997 book *Viral Sex* that science alone cannot control the virus: "Now that the HIV family has found the human family, it will always be with us in some form. All people must know HIV and work to control it" (Goudsmit 1997: 218).

Because there is no immediate hope of curing HIV/AIDS, preventive measures against transmission will remain important into the 21st century. This includes ways to prevent transmission through all infectious body fluids: blood, semen, cervicovaginal secretions and breastmilk.

## Bottle-Feeding Also Risky

In the resource-poor areas of Africa, Asia and Latin America, bottle-feeding is generally unsafe, especially in those areas that still lack clean water and where sanitary conditions are poor. Mothers who cannot afford to buy enough formula dilute it with the only water available to them, which is often unclean. They also feed their babies animal milk or teas, or mixtures of cornstarch and water or flour and water, or whatever semisolid foods are available. All of these, of course, are very poor substitutes for breastmilk. Millions of babies, in fact, have died from inappropriate bottle-feeding, despite the efforts of the World Health Organization and UNICEF, who have been promoting breastfeeding tirelessly for decades. Understandably, breastfeeding advocates fear that if an entire *population* of women give up breastfeeding, even more babies will die. Also, without breastfeeding, women will resume menstruating and ovulating much faster after childbirth, and many would soon become pregnant again. When children are born too soon after their next oldest sibling, they are more likely to die (Hobcraft 1985). Furthermore, mothers of children close in age often lack the financial resources to feed or care for them adequately.

For HIV-negative mothers, there are no alternatives that come close to breastfeeding in providing benefits for babies and mothers. For HIV-positive mothers, alternatives, which need to be appropriate to local conditions, include formula feeding (commercial or generic formula), feeding of animal milks, wet nursing, use of donor breastmilk, heat treatment of breastmilk to inactivate the virus, treatment with drugs and short-term breastfeeding.

## Terms Used with Infant Feeding and HIV

In discussing studies, I will employ the language used by the original researchers. The term "HIV-positive" suggests that someone has had a test for HIV and has tested positive, whereas the term "HIV-infected" accurately describes people who carry the virus but who have not been tested. The term "living with HIV" describes people whose awareness of their seropositivity has an impact on their lives.

Many researchers refer to nonbreastfed babies by the common term "bottle-fed," and I will use the researchers' language, while acknowledging that babies can be "bottle-fed" breastmilk and can be cup-fed formula. I will call infant formula "formula" or "breastmilk substitutes," depending on what the original authors call it. The term "breastmilk substitutes" refers to formula and also to any animal milk or other foods fed to babies as substitutes for breastmilk. I acknowledge that many breastfeeding advocates prefer to call formula "artificial baby milk." Researchers in HIV tend to use the term "bottle-feeding" when referring to nonbreastfed babies. In 1998 a Technical Consultation on HIV and Infant Feeding by the WHO, UNAIDS and UNICEF introduced a new term. "Replacement feeding" means providing a child who receives no breastmilk with a diet that contains all the nutrients that the child needs throughout the period for which breastmilk is recommended — that is, for at least the first two years of life.

I sometimes use the term "Third World" and have come to agree with

Chandra Mohanty (1991: IX) that the contested term "Third World" has a place in referring to anti-imperialist and antiracist struggles.

## HIV Transmission Rates Among
## Breast Versus Bottle-Fed Babies

How likely is it that HIV-infected women transmit the virus to babies whom they breastfeed? Unfortunately, researchers are still unable to provide a definitive answer. When the child of an HIV-infected mother turns out to be HIV-infected also, one does not know whether the child became infected during pregnancy, during the birth process, or through breastfeeding. But by comparing rates of infection between babies who are breastfed and babies who are not, one can get an idea of the additional risk associated with breastfeeding.

In general, the studies on breast and bottle-feeding have found that breastfeeding doubles the risk of HIV transmission. For example, Rubini reported from her research on children in Rio de Janeiro, Brazil, that of children who had been breastfed by HIV-positive mothers, 49.3 percent (37/71) became HIV-infected. Only 18.8 percent (6/32) of the bottle-fed children became infected. These bottle-fed children must have been infected in utero or during the birth process. The breastfed children stood the additional risk attributed to breastfeeding. So, the bottom line, if you will, is that the *bottle-fed* babies of HIV-infected mothers had an approximate 19 percent chance of becoming infected, while *breastfed* babies had an approximate 49 percent chance of being infected. Breastfeeding added an extra 30 percent risk. Breast-fed babies were two and a half times more likely to be infected compared to bottle-fed babies.

Gray (1997), in her research on HIV-positive women in Soweto, South Africa, revealed that the infected mothers had been allowed to choose whether to breast or bottle-feed. There were no significant differences between the breast and bottle-feeders in terms of the demographic data, vaginal or cesarean delivery or CD4 counts (which indicate the relative health of people who are HIV-positive). Gray and colleagues followed the mother-baby pairs for 18 months. Of the children who were breastfed by HIV-positive mothers, 34.6 percent became HIV-infected, compared to 15.5 percent of the formula-fed infants. So, in Soweto also, breastfeeding more than doubled the risk.

Bobat and colleagues (1997) of the University of Natal, South Africa, also concluded that breastfeeding significantly increased the risk of HIV transmission. Thirty-six HIV-positive mothers breastfed exclusively and 39 percent of their babies became HIV-infected. Seventy-six mothers combined breast and formula feeding and 32 percent of their babies became HIV-infected. Twenty-one mothers formula-fed exclusively and 24 percent of their babies became HIV-infected.

Tess (1997, 1998) reported work with 434 HIV-positive mothers in São Paulo, Brazil. Here too breastfeeding more than doubled the risk of a baby's becoming HIV-infected. Tess reported that 264 children were bottle-fed and that 13 percent of them became HIV-infected. Of the 168 children who were breastfed, the risk of infection increased the longer they continued to nurse. Only five (13 percent) of the 38 children who were breastfed for 1–3 days became HIV-infected. Thirty-seven babies were breastfed for at least 91 days, with 11 (30 percent) of them contracting HIV. This finding, that short-term breastfeeding is relatively safe, has been corroborated by other researchers.

Maguire and colleagues (1997) reported that 21 HIV-positive women in Spain had breastfed in the late 1980s, while 450 HIV-positive women had bottle-fed. Of the 21 babies who were breastfed by HIV-positive mothers, 12 (57 percent) became infected, compared to only 76 out of 450 (17 percent) of the bottle-fed babies.

The reports described above are unusual, in that they compared rates of transmission between breast and bottle-fed babies. The vast majority of reports described African populations in which almost all babies are breastfed. I discuss this in the next chapter.

## Older Reports Comparing Transmission Rates Among Breast and Bottle-Fed Babies

The high rates of HIV transmission found in the studies of the mid and late 1990s had been foretold by earlier research. The earlier reports also described a pattern in which breastfed babies were significantly more likely to become HIV-infected than bottle-fed babies. Although the numbers in the early studies were generally small, considered together they suggested years ago that breastfeeding added a significant additional risk.

In 1989, Blanche reported in the *New England Journal of Medicine* that HIV-positive mothers in France were told not to breastfeed and that most mothers complied. Six mothers, however, breastfed against medical advice, and five of their six babies became HIV-infected. Of the 99 babies who were bottle-fed by HIV-positive mothers, only 25 became HIV-infected. So the HIV rates were 83 percent for breastfed babies and 25 percent for bottle-fed babies.

In 1992, Gabiano published results in *Pediatrics*. Among Italian mother-baby pairs in the study, the transmission rate in breastfed babies was 40.9 percent (9/22), compared to 23.2 percent (124/534) in bottle-fed babies.

At the 1992 International Conference on AIDS, Kuznetsova reported that 6 of 23 Soviet mothers had chosen to breastfeed and 5 out of their 6 babies became HIV-infected. The other 17 mothers had chosen to bottle-feed and only one of the 17 babies became HIV-infected. While the numbers of mothers and babies were small, the data reveal that 83 percent of breastfed babies became infected, compared to only 6 percent of the bottle-fed babies. McDonald et al. (1996) reported from Australia that 50 percent (7/14) of breastfed babies became HIV-infected, compared to 17 percent (3/18) of bottle-fed babies.

It should also be noted that two reports from the early 1990s seemed to suggest a negligible difference in the rates of transmission. The breastfed babies in these two reports were HIV-infected at comparatively low rates, similar to the rates among bottle-fed babies.

Halsey and colleagues (1990) in Haiti found that breastfed babies of HIV-positive mothers were infected at a rate of approximately 25 percent. They described this as being similar to reports among bottle-fed babies in the United States and Europe. But, as Halsey noted, they may have had an "artificially low estimate of HIV-1 transmission" because many of the babies living under the worst conditions of poverty were unavailable for follow-up.

Semba's 1994 report from Malawi focused largely on vitamin A, but it also noted the rates of HIV transmission among the babies, all of whom were breastfed. When children who died in the first year were excluded from analysis, the rate of HIV transmission was only 21.9 percent. But when they included the data from the babies who died early, the overall rate of HIV transmission was 35.1 percent.

## A Meta-Analysis Based Largely on Short-Term Breastfeeding

In 1992, Dunn and colleagues published a meta-analysis using the best early data that were available. They concluded that among mothers who were HIV-infected prior to the pregnancy, the children stand a 14 percent greater risk of contracting the virus as a result of breastfeeding. Dunn also concluded that women who become newly HIV-infected while they are breastfeeding have an additional 29 percent risk of transmitting HIV to their children.

In one of the six studies analyzed by Dunn, the duration was typical of the prolonged breastfeeding found in resource-poor countries. That one report was Ryder's report from Zaire (now renamed the Democratic Republic of Congo). Ryder noted that affluent women in Zaire prefer to bottle-feed. None (0 percent) of the 10 exclusively bottle-fed babies of HIV-positive mothers became HIV-infected, compared to 20 percent of the 28 exclusively breastfed babies.

The other five studies analyzed by Dunn had been conducted in the United States, Switzerland, Europe, France and Australia. Durations of breastfeeding in these five reports were brief: two weeks, less than four weeks, four weeks, seven weeks and two weeks to nine months. In Kind's 1992 report from

Switzerland, 13 babies were breastfed for about two weeks. Only 2 out of 13 (15 percent) breastfed babies became infected. This was very close in risk to the 16 percent infection rate among 128 bottle-fed babies.

Hutto (1991) had reported data about 25 babies in Miami, Florida, who were breastfed briefly. The duration was not recorded, but all mothers — as of four weeks after delivery — were told not to breastfeed. In this group, the breastfed babies were actually less likely to be infected, as 28 percent (7/25) of the breastfed babies contracted the virus, compared to 33 percent (18/54) of the bottle-fed babies. Why such a large percentage of the bottle-fed babies became HIV-infected is not clear. They may have been born to mothers with relatively advanced HIV disease.

The French data, as used in an updated version, revealed that 44 percent (7/16) of the breastfed babies were infected, compared to 17 percent (101/590) of the bottle-fed babies. The Australian data supplied to Dunn showed that 50 percent (7/14) of the breastfed babies became infected, compared to 17 percent (3/18) of the bottle-fed babies. From the European Collaborative Study (1992) came the report that 41 HIV-positive mothers had breastfed their babies for a median duration of four weeks. In this group, 32 percent (13/41) of the breastfed babies became infected, compared to only 14 percent (110/767) of the bottle-fed babies.

Dunn's widely quoted 14 percent figure (that is, the risk attributable to breastfeeding over and above the risk of transmission through birth) was calculated based on information available in 1992, which was prior to the publication of studies emphasizing the importance of duration.

Later meta-analyses found that the risk associated with breastfeeding was greater than 14 percent. According to one meta-analysis, the risk associated with short-term breastfeeding is 11 percent, while for long-term breastfeeding the risk jumps to 24 percent (John 1997). This finding is of grave concern because long-term breastfeeding is the common pattern in resource-poor countries.

Nieburg and Stanecki (1998) noted that one more recent meta-analysis found that the risk associated with breastfeeding for more than three months is 21 percent. They noted that the 1997 UNAIDS figure may underestimate the true pediatric HIV disease burden and that much of the potential underestimate is associated with transmission through breastfeeding. Of the 2,032,000 births expected to occur to HIV-infected women in 1998, 406,000 (20 percent) will be infected in either the intrauterine or intrapartum periods. The number of babies infected through breastfeeding would be as low as 273,000 if breastfeeding contributed only a 14 percent additional risk, or as high as 410,000 if breastfeeding contributed an additional 21 percent risk. They concluded that breastmilk transmission of HIV could account for as much as 50 percent of all mother-to-child transmission.

## An Overview of the Breast Versus Bottle Rates

The overall rates of HIV transmission from HIV-infected mothers to their breast and bottle-fed children are noted below:

| Country, Researcher | Bottle-fed, percentage infected | Breastfed, percentage infected |
|---|---|---|
| Brazil, Rubini | 19 | 49 |
| South Africa, Gray | 15 | 35 |
| South Africa, Bobat | 24 | 39 |
| Spain, Maguire | 17 | 57 |
| France, Blanche | 25 | 83 |
| Italy, Gabiano | 23 | 41 |
| Russia, Kuznetsova | 6 | 83 |
| Australia, McDonald | 17 | 50 |
| Zaire, Ryder | 0 | 20 |
| Switzerland, Kind | 16 | 15 |
| USA, Hutto | 33 | 28 |
| European Collab. | 14 | 32 |

## References

Ammann, Arthur J. 1997. Setting worldwide goals for reducing transmission from mothers to infants. Presented at the Conference on Global Strategies for the Prevention of HIV Transmission from Mothers to Infants, Washington, D.C., September 3–6.

Blanche, S., et al. 1989. A prospective study of perinatal infection of infants born to women seropositive for human immunodeficiency virus type 1. *New England Journal of Medicine* 320: 1643–1648.

Bobat, R., Moodley Dhayendree, Anna Coutsoudis and Hoosen Coovadia. 1997. Breastfeeding by HIV-1-infected women and outcome in their infants: A cohort study from Durban, South Africa. *AIDS* 11: 1627–1633.

Centers for Disease Control and Prevention. 1985. Recommendations for assisting in the prevention of perinatal transmission of human T-lymphotropic virus type III/lymphaedeonopathy. *Morbidity and Mortality Weekly Report* 34: 721–732.

_____. 1998. Vertical transmission rates may be higher than predicted. *Reuters News Service*, July 23.

Dunn, D. T., M. L. Newell, A. E. Ades, and C. S. Peckham. 1992. Risk of human immunodeficiency virus type 1 transmission through breastfeeding. *Lancet* 340: 585–588.

European Collaborative Study. 1992. Risk factors for mother-to-child transmission of HIV-1. *Lancet* 339: 1007–1012.

Gabiano, Clara, et al. 1992. Mother-to-child transmission of HIV type 1: Risk of infection and correlates of transmission. *Pediatrics* 90: 69–74.

Goudsmit, J. 1997. *Viral Sex: The Nature of AIDS*. New York/Oxford: Oxford University Press.

Gray, Glenda E. 1997. Breastfeeding-related transmission. Presented at the Fourth International Conference on AIDS in Asia and the Pacific, Manila, Philippines, October 25–29. Abstract FA10.

Halsey, Neal A., et al. 1990. Transmission of HIV-1 infections from mothers to infants in Haiti. *Journal of the American Medical Association* 264: 2088–2092.

Health Ministry (of Brazil) PN DST/AIDS. 1995. *Breast-feeding versus HIV-infected Women Recommendations*.

Hobcraft, J. N., J. W. McDonald and S. O. Rutstein. 1985. Demographic determinants of infant and early child mortality: A comparative analysis. *Population Studies* 39: 363–385.

Hutto, C., et al. 1991. A hospital-based prospective study of perinatal infection with human immunodeficiency virus type 1. *Journal of Pediatrics* 118: 347–353.

John, G. 1997. Epidemiology of HIV-1 transmission through breastfeeding. Presented at the Conference on Affordable Options for the Prevention of Mother-to-Child Transmission of HIV-1, Johannesburg, South Africa, November 19–20.

Kind, C., et al. 1992. Epidemiology of vertically transmitted HIV-1 infection in Switzerland: Results of a nationwide prospective study. *European Journal of Pediatrics* 151: 442–448.

Kuznetsova, I., et al. 1992. Prevention of maternal infant HIV-transmission by weaning. Presented at the Eighth International Conference on AIDS, Amsterdam, Netherlands, July 19–24.

Luzuriaga, Katherine, and John J. Sullivan. 1998. Prevention and treatment of pediatric HIV infection. *Journal of the American Medical Association* 280: 17–18.

Maguire, A., et al. 1997. Potential risk factors for vertical HIV-1 transmission in Catalonia, Spain: The protective role of Cesarean section. *AIDS* 11: 1851–1857.

McDonald, A., et al. 1996. Perinatal exposure to HIV in Australia, 1982–1995. Presented at the Annual Conference by Australia's Society for HIV Medicine, November 14–17.

Mohanty, Chandra Talpede. 1991. *Third World Women and the Politics of Feminism*. Bloomington, Indiana: Indiana University Press.

National AIDS Programme and the Perinatal HIV Research Unit. 1997. Presented at the Conference on Affordable Options for the Prevention of Mother-to-Child Transmission of HIV-1, Johannesburg, South Africa, November 19–20.

Nieburg, Phillip and K. A. Stanecki. 1998. The global burden of mother-to-child transmission of HIV-1. Presented at the Twelfth World AIDS Conference, Geneva, Switzerland, June 28–July 3, Abstract 13591.

Piot, Peter. 1997. Fighting AIDS together. In *The Progress of Nations 1997*. New York: UNICEF.

Rubini, N. P. M., et. al. 1996. HIV vertical transmission in Rio de Janeiro: Rate and risk factors. Presented at the Eleventh International Conference on AIDS, Vancouver, Canada, July 7–12. Abstract Tu.C.2570.

Ryder, R. W., et al. 1991. Evidence from Zaire that breast-feeding by HIV-1-seropositive mothers is not a major route for perinatal HIV-1 transmission but does decrease morbidity. *AIDS* 5: 709–714.

Semba, Richard D., et al. 1994. Maternal vitamin A deficiency and mother-to-child transmission of HIV-1. *Lancet* 343: 1593–1597.

Tess, B. H., L. C. Rodrigues, M.-L. Newell and D. T. Dunn. 1997. Risk factors for mother-to-infant transmission of HIV-1 in São Paulo State, Brazil. Presented at the Fourth Conference on Retroviruses and Opportunistic Infections, Washington, D.C., January 22–27.

Tess, Beatriz H., et al. 1998. Breastfeeding, genetic, obstetric and other risk factors associated with mother-to-child transmission of HIV-1 in São Paulo State, Brazil. *AIDS* 12: 513–520.

UNAIDS. 1997a. *Best Practice Collection Point of View: The Female Condom and HIV/AIDS*. Geneva, Switzerland: UNAIDS.

_____. 1997b. *Breastfeeding and HIV/AIDS*. Geneva, Switzerland: UNAIDS.

_____. 1997c. *HIV and Infant Feeding*. A Policy Statement. Geneva, Switzerland: UNAIDS.

_____. 1997d. *Report on the Global HIV/AIDS Epidemic*. Geneva, Switzerland: UNAIDS.

_____. 1998. International meeting calls for concerted action to prevent mother-to-child transmission of HIV. Press release, Geneva, Switzerland, March 24.

UNAIDS Joint United Nations Programme on HIV/AIDS. 1996. HIV and infant feeding: An interim statement. *Weekly Epidemiological Record* 71: 289–291.

World Health Organization. 1987. Breast-feeding/breast milk and human immunodeficiency virus (HIV). *Weekly Epidemiological Record* 33: 245–246.

World Health Organization Global Programme on AIDS. 1992. Consensus statement from the WHO/UNICEF Constitution on HIV transmission and breast feeding. *Weekly Epidemiological Record*. 67: 177–184.

CHAPTER TWO

---

# Fourteen Years of
# Research Showing That
# Breastmilk Transmits HIV

Research conducted in populations, mostly African, in which almost all babies of HIV-infected mothers were breastfed is discussed in this chapter. Although these reports do not lend themselves to direct "breast versus bottle" comparisons, they offer much insight into the phenomenon of HIV transmission through breastmilk.

The first report published in a medical journal was the 1985 report by Australian physician John Ziegler. An Australian woman breastfed after becoming HIV-infected by a postpartum transfusion of blood, later traced to a man with AIDS. She did not know that she had been infected when she breastfed her baby, who was later diagnosed as having AIDS. It seemed highly likely that she had transmitted the virus via breastfeeding. Ziegler's report alerted the world to the possibility of HIV transmission through breastmilk.

Other reports also presented the case histories of women who breastfed after being transfused with HIV-infected blood. Reports came from Australia (Palasanthiran 1993), France (Weinbreck 1988), India (Malaviya 1992), Mexico (Flores 1991), Rwanda (Lepage 1987), the United States (Stiehm 1991), Zaire (Colebunders 1988), and Zambia (Hira 1990). The encouraging news from some of these early reports was that many babies who were breastfed by newly infected women escaped infection. Ziegler joined with other Australian colleagues, including lead author Pamela Palasanthiran (1993), to

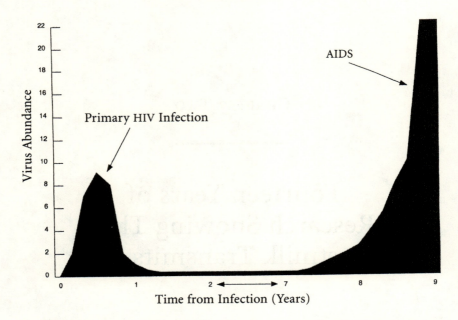

**Variable viremia over the incubation period of AIDS. Reproduced from *AIDS in the World II* with permission of Dr. Daniel Tarantola.**

report that, of eleven Australian babies who were breastfed by transfusion-infected mothers, only three became HIV-infected. Colebunders (1988) reported that three women in Zaire received HIV-infected blood transfusions but that only one of the babies breastfed by these three mothers became HIV-infected. Colebunders also described the case of HIV transmission by a wet nurse in Zaire. The woman was dying from AIDS when she wet-nursed her nephew and apparently transmitted the virus to the child, who also died from AIDS.

It is now known that people are very infectious when their HIV disease has developed into full-blown AIDS. People are also quite infectious in the months just after they become HIV-infected (Daar 1991), when they are first seroconverting from HIV-negative to HIV-positive. At these times, after the onset of AIDS or in the weeks following seroconversion, the amount of virus in the blood, or "viral load," is high. The transfusion-infected mothers, who were breastfeeding at the time of seroconversion, were likely to have been highly infectious; nevertheless, many of the babies escaped infection. The figure above shows the virus abundance over the time from infection in years.

## Detecting the Virus in Breastmilk

Thiry's 1985 report supported the idea that HIV could be transmitted via breastmilk. In five milk samples from three HIV-positive African women, Thiry isolated the AIDS virus from cell-free breastmilk. Later reports also confirmed that the virus was detected in breastmilk. What Thiry referred to as the "AIDS virus" had been identified as HIV in 1983 and was later declared HIV-1.

Van de Perre and colleagues (1988) reported that they had found HIV antibodies in all milk specimens from four HIV-positive mothers in Rwanda; in three out of four cases, the babies were also HIV-positive. Ruff and colleagues (1994) reported that they found HIV DNA in 70 percent of samples collected from women zero to four days postpartum, and in 50 percent of milk samples collected from women six to twelve months postpartum.

Nduati and other colleagues (1995) in Nairobi, Kenya, studied 212 breastmilk samples, collected at varying times after delivery, from 107 HIV-positive women. They found that as of nine months after delivery 58 percent of samples of breastmilk had detectable HIV-1-infected cells. In contrast to previous studies, Nduati found a significantly higher prevalence of HIV in mature milk than in colostrum (early milk). Women with more advanced HIV disease and women with severe vitamin A deficiency were more likely to have HIV in their milk. Nduati concluded that most HIV-positive women shed infected cells, and that a breastfed baby might ingest hundreds of thousands of HIV-infected cells per day. Colostrum contains a higher concentration of cells (macrophages and lymphocytes) than mature milk and may be more likely to harbor cell-associated HIV.

Breastmilk has been nicknamed "white blood" because, like blood, it contains cells associated with the immune system. The macrophages, lymphocytes and other cells in breastmilk are usually protective for the immature human infant, but not so with HIV.

In 1998 Lewis, Nduati and other colleagues in Nairobi found that the prevalence of cell-free HIV-1 was higher in mature milk (47 percent) than in colostrum (27 percent). Thus withholding colostrum (i.e., not starting breastfeeding until a few days after birth) would not protect babies, as once was thought. The risk of transmission is likely to be related to, among other factors, the quantity of HIV-1 in cell-free breastmilk and the number of HIV-1-infected cells. It is not known whether women with compromised immune systems produce milk that is different from that produced by women with normal immune systems.

## HIV-1, HIV-2, HIV-0

During the time of initial reports about breastfeeding and HIV, it was assumed that there was one virus, commonly referred to as "HIV" for "Human

Immunodeficiency Virus." In 1985 a second virus, HIV-2, was recognized. While HIV-1 is found in almost every country on earth, HIV-2 has been limited to West Africa and India, and to people who have had contact with those regions. HIV-2 accounts for less than 1 percent of all HIV infections. A third virus, HIV-0, was identified in 1990 in Cameroon and Gabon. HIV-0, however, is rare even in those countries, and little is known about it.

Prior exposure to the less virulent HIV-2 strain may provide protection against HIV-1 infection (Travers 1998). People who are HIV-2-infected progress to symptomatic disease much more slowly than people who are HIV-1-infected. The modes of transmission are the same, but HIV-2 is less readily transmitted sexually or from mother to child. Marlink (1997) concluded that while HIV-1-infected mothers transmit the virus to their children in 25–35 percent of cases, HIV-2-infected mothers transmit in 0–4 percent of cases.

Among children born to *HIV-1-positive* mothers in The Gambia, 17/79 (21.5 percent) were HIV-positive at age 18 months (O'Donovan 1997). For children born to *HIV-2-positive* mothers, only 9/194 (4.6 percent) became infected. Of these nine, three did not become HIV-2-infected until after nine months, which suggests that they were likely HIV-2-infected through breastfeeding in the later months. A subsequent report from this same research cohort noted that maternal HIV-1 infection and especially maternal death significantly increased the risk of child mortality even among uninfected children (Ota 1998).

## Other Viruses Spread in Milk

Most common viruses, in any species of mammal, are not spread by mother's milk. The conventional wisdom is that a breastfeeding mother should keep nursing while she is suffering from, for instance, the common cold. That way, the antibodies she makes will appear in her milk and will lessen the severity of the symptoms should her baby catch the cold. Another reason for continuing breastfeeding with most viruses comes from the probability that, by the time the mother realizes she is infected, the baby would already be exposed to the virus.

Although most viruses are not spread in breastmilk, a few are. In general, retroviruses are most readily transmitted in milk. Many retroviruses found in animals are readily transmitted by mother's milk. One retrovirus, capine arthritis-encephalitis virus (CAEV), found in goats is so readily transmissible that, when goat's milk is pooled to feed many kid goats, the milk from one CAEV-infected mother goat can infect almost all kids who feed on the pooled milk (Adams 1984).

Breastfeeding is believed to be a major mode of transmission for the first human retrovirus to be isolated, human T-cell leukemia virus type-I

(HTLV-I) (Hino 1985). Also transmitted through sexual contact, blood trans-fusions and needle sharing, HTLV-I is linked with the development of adult T-cell leukemia. The retrovirus is clustered in Japan (around Nagasaki), in the Caribbean and in parts of Africa and South America. Pregnant women in Nagasaki are now screened, and if they carry HTLV-I they are told not to breast-feed (Kawase 1992).

Much less is known about HTLV-II, which has been found in certain African and Native American populations and among intravenous drug users. Heneine and colleagues from the CDC reported in 1992 that they had detected HTLV-II in 83.3 percent of the samples of breastmilk from Panamanian Indian women who were infected with this virus; they found none of the samples of milk from noninfected women (Heneine 1992). Although little is known about HTLV-II, it is believed to be transmitted through breastfeeding (Kaplan 1992), and the CDC (1993) has recommended that women infected with HTLV-II not breastfeed.

Caterino-De-Araulo (1998) noted that among 107 nonbreastfed children in São Paulo, none became infected with HTLV-I or HTLV-II.

## Cytomegalovirus and HIV

Cytomegalovirus (CMV) is another virus that is transmitted via breast-milk. While CMV transmission via breastmilk is common, it produces no ill effects in most babies. Extremely immature infants, however, face symptomatic CMV infection. Vochem and colleagues found that the transmission rate was 59 percent among preemies fed breastmilk from CMV-positive mothers. The researchers recommended pasteurizing or freezing breastmilk from CMV-pos-itive mothers of extremely immature infants.

Some babies who are coinfected with HIV and CMV are at increased risk of symptomatic CMV infection because of compromised immune function (Mussi-Pinhata 1998). This is an important concern because there is a very high prevalence of CMV infection among HIV-infected persons. In Mussi-Pinhata's study, 94 percent of babies of HIV-infected mothers in Brazil were not breastfed, so few (only 7.9 percent) experienced perinatal CMV infections. Infections were termed "perinatal" if they were detected after four weeks of age. "Congenital" infection happened earlier and could be detected shortly after birth.

But most babies of HIV-negative mothers were breastfed, and 39 percent experienced perinatal CMV infection. Nevertheless, the perinatal CMV infec-tion among HIV-negative babies was asymptomatic, except for two of the thirteen babies, who had minor symptoms. Of eight HIV-infected, CMV-infected mothers who had not transmitted CMV earlier, four transmitted CMV later, very likely via breastmilk.

Black (1996) of the United States suggested that HIV-infected mothers consider breastfeeding infants who are already HIV-infected themselves. But Mussi-Pinhata's study suggests an additional consideration. If an HIV-infected mother is coinfected with CMV, she might transmit it to a baby who was previously HIV-infected but CMV-uninfected. In that case, the possible benefits of breastmilk could be negated by symptomatic CMV infection in an immuno-compromised baby. If an HIV-positive woman in an industrialized country were considering breastfeeding a baby who was already HIV-infected, she would need medical advice about her own CMV status and that of the baby.

## Other Early Reports About HIV Transmission

While reports from 1985 (Ziegler and Thiry) suggested that HIV was transmitted in breastmilk, it was hoped that breastfeeding was an uncommon mode of transmission. In the early and mid–1980s, no one knew when or how babies became HIV-infected. Outside of research centers, African mothers were not tested, nor are most of them to this day. The "diagnosis" might be made by observing that someone died with symptoms consistent with AIDS. But symptoms that are consistent with AIDS (diarrhea, respiratory problems) are also found with other common diseases. When a child in a resource-poor country has diarrhea, the cause of it is usually not known.

To make a diagnosis, or to conduct HIV research, it is obviously crucial to know the person's HIV status. The commonly used HIV tests, the ELISA (Enzyme-Linked ImmunoSorbent Assay) and Western Blot, screen blood for the presence of HIV antibodies — not for the virus itself. It takes several weeks or even longer after infection before antibodies can be detected in the blood.

Testing newborn babies for antibodies is particularly problematic. If the mother is HIV-antibody-positive, her baby will be HIV-antibody-positive for a time. All newborns born to HIV-positive mothers will test antibody-positive because the test will detect the mother's antibodies in the baby's blood. Maternal antibodies often persist for up to 15 months, occasionally for even longer. But tests that identify the virus itself — rather than antibodies to the virus — are accurate fairly early after infection. The polymerase chain reaction (PCR), which tests for the presence of the virus, may be able to diagnose HIV infection in babies at two weeks of age (Krivine 1997). But before four weeks of age, there may not be enough virus in the baby's bloodstream for accurate PCR testing.

The earliest research on transmission of HIV via breastmilk was conducted in the era when the only HIV tests available were antibody tests. Using these antibody tests, researchers could not tell if babies were or were not infected in the early months. Researchers convened in Ghent, Belgium, and agreed to use 15 months of age as the cutoff point for determining a baby's HIV status (Dabis 1992).

There had been reports of babies who appeared to be HIV-positive early on, but who later tested negative. This suggested that some babies might have transient HIV infections that cleared. But when researchers reanalyzed the HIV tests, they found no cases that satisfied the criteria for transient infection. Most of the conflicting test results, it was decided, resulted from lab errors, the product of mishandling or contamination of the samples (Frenkel 1998).

Researchers have long sought to understand why some babies of HIV-1-positive mothers became infected while others did not. In their attempts to understand what protected some infants, a few researchers first focused on the possible role of antibodies in breastmilk. Van de Perre and colleagues (1988) found HIV antibodies in the milk of all four HIV-positive breastfeeding women. But the antibodies in the milk were not protective. Three out of the four babies became infected, despite their mothers' antibodies. Van de Perre (1993) later reported that the presence in milk of one of the immunoglobulins, IgM, was associated with a lower risk of transmission. Researchers could now predict how likely it was for the child of an HIV-1-positive mother to become infected. The mother who had more HIV-1-infected cells in her milk and a defective IgM response was most likely to infect her child (Van de Perre 1993).

Bélec and colleagues (1990) reported that they had examined antibodies to HIV-1 in the breastmilk of 15 asymptomatic HIV-1-positive women in the Central African Republic. It had been *hypothesized* that the antibodies to HIV (in blood, semen, vaginal secretions and milk) might limit transmission. But some of the babies became HIV-infected despite the presence of maternal antibodies in breastmilk.

Duprat and colleagues (1994) reported that they had examined HIV-1 antibodies, called anti-HIV-1 secretory IgA, in the breastmilk and blood of women in Nairobi, Kenya. Fifty-nine percent of HIV-positive mothers did have the antibodies in their breastmilk. The secretory IgA, however, did not protect the babies from the HIV virus. This was surprising because secretory IgA is a major protective factor against *other* diseases.

Researchers such as Hira (1989), Lallemant (1994), and Tess (1998) reported that mothers who were most symptomatic were more likely to transmit the virus than those who were less symptomatic. Tess reported that Brazilian mothers with advanced maternal HIV-1 disease were more than four times as likely to transmit as healthier mothers.

Hira's 1989 observation that some babies' HIV antibody test results go from positive to negative to positive again was eventually corroborated. A few years later, researchers in Kenya (Datta 1994), the Congo (Lallemant 1994), Rwanda (Bulterys 1995), Zaire (Bertolli 1996) and Côte d'Ivoire (Ekpini 1997) also reported that children were HIV-negative for months before becoming

HIV-positive again, apparently through breastfeeding. It is now recognized that neonates born to HIV-infected mothers will first test antibody-positive because of maternal antibodies. But many will have escaped becoming HIV-infected before or during birth and will test antibody negative for several months. Later some of these babies will test positive again if they have become HIV-infected through breastmilk.

## Women Who Experience a Primary HIV Infection During Breastfeeding

By 1990–1991, researchers were reporting that women who seroconvert while breastfeeding are the most likely to transmit the virus to their breast-feeding children. Of 634 Zambian women who were HIV-negative when they gave birth, 19 became HIV-infected during the months of breastfeeding (Hira 1990). Of these 19, three had babies who also became HIV-infected. Hira suggested that women at high risk of acquiring HIV, particularly those who have sexual relationships with HIV-infected men, be advised not to breastfeed, though only if the region's mortality/morbidity risk is not significant.

Van de Perre and colleagues (1991) also described women who were HIV-negative when they started breastfeeding but who later became infected. In their study, 210 mothers were HIV-1-negative when they gave birth. Of the 210 women, 16 became HIV-1-infected while they were breastfeeding, probably via sexual contact. Of these 16 women, nine had babies who also became HIV-1-infected, always during the same three months in which the mothers became infected.

The cases in Rwanda (Van de Perre 1991) and Zambia (Hira 1990) of women who became infected sexually were similar to the early reports of women who were infected via blood transfusions and who then breastfed. In both circumstances, women were breastfeeding during the time of primary infection. As of 1988, most — although not all — blood is screened; so one would not expect so many women to be HIV-infected by transfusion around the time they breastfeed. Heterosexual transmission, however, is rapidly increasing. Women who become HIV-1-positive after they begin breastfeeding stand a great risk of infecting their breastfeeding children. It has been estimated that 10 percent of *all infant mortality* in South Africa can be attributed to breastfeeding by women who become HIV-infected while breastfeeding (*Affordable Options* 1997).

## Breast/Nipple Problems as Increased Risks

In 1992 Van de Perre and colleagues reported that the risk of transmission increased if the mother experienced a breast abscess. They described the case of one of the women from the Rwandan group. She became HIV-infected, twelve months after delivery, while still breastfeeding.

Although this mother continued to breastfeed her child during and after her primary infection, the child remained HIV-1-negative, by PCR and Western Blot, for more than a year. It was not until the mother developed a severe breast abscess, at month 28, that she apparently transmitted the virus to her child through breastfeeding. She required surgical treatment for the breast abscess and stopped breastfeeding one week after suppuration. When her child was tested at age 30 months and at age 36 months, he was HIV-1-positive by PCR and Western Blot.

Van de Perre's case history suggested that HIV-1 can be transmitted during breastfeeding more than one year after the mother's primary infection. He felt that the breast abscess was associated with inflammatory cells, which the child ingested. Van de Perre suggested that, if his observation was confirmed, HIV-1-infected mothers should abandon breastfeeding as soon as a breast abscess develops, especially with older children.

Van de Perre noted that this additional case brought the risk of postnatal transmission, among newly infected breastfeeding women, to between 45 and 60 percent, depending on whether one counted a single infection that happened in the first three months of an infant's life. In such instances, infection may have occurred during birth or during early breastfeeding.

Njenga and colleagues (1997) from Kenya noted that thrush in babies' mouths also increases the risk of infection by breastfeeding. Babies who had oral thrush before they were six months old were almost three times more likely to become HIV-infected. These researchers believe that oral thrush increases the chance of a baby's becoming infected, since it causes breaks in the mucosal barrier of the baby's mouth. Thrush is extremely common and may be present even without visual signs (Hoover 1997).

Opperman (1997) reported that in Zimbabwe breastfeeding mothers who had nipple problems were more likely to infect their babies. She also reported that babies who had had oral disease were more likely to become HIV-infected. In Karlsson's (1997) report from Tanzania, however, none of the mothers who transmitted HIV to their toddlers reported any breast or nipple problems.

## Case Histories of Older Children

Case histories describing HIV transmission via breastfeeding to older children are especially instructive in that they describe women's actual infant feeding practices, which often differ from official recommendations. No one recommends, for instant, that a mother pass up nursing her newborn baby to nurse her 2-year-old child. But this happened in a case history reported by Rubini and colleagues (1992). A Brazilian mother gave birth to children in

1979, 1981 and 1983. After her second delivery, in 1981, the mother received two transfusions of blood. The infant was premature and did not nurse well. The mother opted to nurse not her new baby but rather her 2-year-old daughter, continuing to do so for several months.

Five years later, in 1986, the mother was ill and was diagnosed as HIV-positive. Then in 1991, the oldest child was ill and was also diagnosed with HIV. The father and two younger siblings remained well and HIV-negative. The family had no apparent risk factors other than the blood transfusion. It seems likely that the mother was infected via the transfusion and the oldest child by breastfeeding.

Rubini noted that this case was distinct in that it involved an older child. She was 24 months old at the time she nursed alongside her newborn sister, who, having breastfed only briefly, was HIV-negative at age 10 years. The infected child breastfed for several months when she was between 2 and 3 years old. The third child, born in 1983, risked HIV infection in utero and during birth as well as during breastfeeding. But she was also HIV-negative at age 8 years. The only factor peculiar to the case of the infected child is one of timing: she breastfed during the time of initial infection and continued for several months.

Datta and colleagues (1992) also reported a case of apparent transmission of HIV to an older child. An HIV-positive Kenyan woman delivered a healthy baby in 1986. The mother breastfed him for seven months and then weaned him because she was pregnant again. Medical problems arose, however, and the second pregnancy was terminated. She then resumed breastfeeding the first child, who was then 11 months old, continuing until the child was 25 months of age, when she was pregnant again. After the birth of the next child, the mother breastfed the new baby and also resumed nursing the older child. She nursed both children for 18 months.

When the mother became ill with symptoms consistent with AIDS, all family members were tested. The youngest child was found to be HIV-positive at 18 months of age. The oldest child presents an unusual case history. He was HIV-antibody-positive at birth, presumably because of the presence of maternal antibodies. So the mother apparently was HIV-positive but appeared healthy at the time of the first child's birth in 1986. This same child had been tested at ages 12 and 18 months by PCR and was HIV-negative. Later testing suggested that he had become HIV-infected by the time he was almost 4 years old. Datta noted that this child appeared to have escaped perinatal infection, as he was HIV-negative at 12 and 18 months of age, according to PCR testing. At age 18 months, however, an immunoblot test revealed bands that four months earlier hadn't appeared, suggesting that infection may have occurred shortly before the age of 44 months.

Apparently this child escaped infection at birth and through early breastfeeding; at the time of his birth his mother had a lower risk of transmitting

HIV. But as the mother's HIV disease progressed, she became more infectious. Thus she likely infected him when she resumed breastfeeding. The mother was following a cultural practice of resuming breastfeeding to help ease the insecurity of the child who was displaced from being the baby of the family.

Avila (1997) reported the case of an Argentinean mother who was originally HIV-negative but whose husband was HIV-positive. Mother and baby were both negative at the child's birth and at ten months after the birth. The mother breastfed the child for 24 months. When at 32 months old he manifested symptoms consistent with AIDS, she took him to an outpatient clinic, where both mother and child tested HIV-positive. The mother appears to have become HIV-infected through sex some time between 10 and 32 months postpartum and then transmitted the virus in her milk. Avila noted that HIV-positive women in Argentina are strongly dissuaded from breastfeeding, but she believes that women at high risk for becoming infected should also be informed of the potential for HIV transmission via breastmilk.

## Hypothesis About Delayed Progression to AIDS

In a 1990 letter to the editor of the journal *AIDS*, Italian physician Alberto Tozzi hypothesized that HIV-1-infected infants who are breastfed may progress more slowly to AIDS than HIV-infected infants who are formula-fed. Tozzi acknowledged in his letter that, by 5 years of age, the rates of developing AIDS were the same. Tozzi suggested that factors in breastmilk might keep HIV-positive children healthier longer, as seemed to be the case with his research subjects, a cohort of Italian children. Tozzi did not disclose whether the Italian women who breast or formula-fed were equally matched in terms of their viral load or strain of HIV. Nor did he indicate whether the Italian women who selected to breastfeed were feeling any better than the HIV-infected women who chose not to breastfeed.

Later reports about the same cohort of Italian children failed to support Tozzi's hypothesis. Tovo (1994) reported that the speed with which children progressed to disease depended on the speed with which their mothers progressed, suggesting that speed is affected by the strain of virus or genetic factors that mother and child share. De Martino (1994a) later reported that the long-term and short-term survival rates in this Italian cohort did not differ, regardless of whether they had been breast or formula-fed.

Frederick (1997), however, presented data that showed that breastfed children progressed more slowly to AIDS. The cases in this report developed between 1988 and 1996 in Los Angeles, California. Some women were not aware that they were HIV-infected, and 43 percent (60/138) of them breastfed their children. Median time to AIDS was 42 months for nonbreastfed children and 74 months for breastfed children (Frederick 1997).

Tozzi's hypothesis, however, was not supported by work in South Africa (Bobat 1997). Among HIV-1-infected children, progression to AIDS was not significantly delayed by breastfeeding. In 20 months of study, none of the HIV-infected formula-fed children progressed to AIDS, while 50 percent of the exclusively breastfed children did. Of the children who were fed both breastmilk and formula, 54 percent developed AIDS.

The children who progress to AIDS faster (i.e., the formula-fed children) may do so because they were infected earlier. Since these children were not breastfed, they must have been HIV-infected before or during birth, and may have had mothers with more advanced HIV disease. Bobat and colleagues noted that they could not assess whether differences in the rate of progression to AIDS were due to dissimilarities in the proportions of babies infected in utero, during delivery or via breastfeeding.


## Reports About the Duration of Breastfeeding

A number of researchers have reported that the longer an HIV-1-positive woman breastfeeds, the more likely she is to transmit the virus to her child (De Martino 1992, Datta 1994, Bertolli 1996, Tess 1997, Ekpini 1997, Macdonald 1998). De Martino and colleagues first reported this phenomenon based on their evaluation of 168 Italian children who were breastfed by HIV-1-positive mothers, and 793 children who were exclusively bottle-fed. One day of breastfeeding added very little additional risk; the odds were only 1.19 times greater for a child breastfed one day, compared to a child who never went to breast. But children who were breastfed for a median duration of two months were 2.7 times more likely to become HIV-1-infected than bottle-fed children. All children enrolled in the Italian Register were born to women with documented HIV-1 infection at delivery, including children who were enrolled retrospectively, after delivery (De Martino and Tovo 1993).

Nagelkerke and colleagues in Nairobi, Kenya, first suggested that breastfeeding for three to seven months might balance the benefits and risks of breastfeeding by HIV-1-infected mothers in resource-poor countries (1995). Datta (1994) reported that they continued to retest the Nairobi children even after the children's earlier test results at twelve or eighteen months were HIV-negative. The testing suggested that some children acquired HIV infection after twelve to eighteen months, most likely from breastfeeding. Of the 90 infected children, 40 had been antibody-negative for approximately six months. These 40 probably acquired their infection from breastfeeding after twelve to eighteen months of age. Previously, some research teams had discontinued testing once a child had a negative HIV test result. It is now recommended that researchers continue to follow children for three months after they are weaned from the breast.

Macdonald (1998) reported in a study nested in the Nairobi research that the mean age when older babies seroconverted to positive was 13 months. There appear to be times when infection via breastfeeding is more likely to occur, although possible risk factors such as breaks in the skin with teething or changing immunologic function are not clearly understood.

Taha and colleges (1995) reported results of a study of infected mothers in urban Malawi. The mother-to-child transmission rate was 35.1 percent. Babies were screened at one year or later. Taha and colleagues (1998) later reported that of 621 originally HIV-negative babies, 47 babies converted to positive between 8 and 18 weeks, 11 converted between 19 and 60 weeks, and 23 converted after 60 weeks. The researchers did not count the 42 conversions that happened between birth and 7 weeks, as these could have been due to infection during birth (or early breastfeeding). Taha, like Hira, suggested that mothers be advised to bottle-feed only if the risk of transmission via breast-feeding is greater than the mortality/morbidity risk of not breastfeeding.

Bulterys (1995) reported the case of six Rwandan children who were anti-body negative by 12 months of age. Four children became HIV-positive at age 28 months and two by 36 months of age. Bulterys reported that all six sero-converting children were breastfed for at least 24 months.

Other researchers also reported that breastfeeding beyond 12 or 24 months had a stronger association with HIV-1-infection. Working in the Republic of Congo, Lallemant and colleagues (1994) observed that the overall transmission rate from mother to child was 40.4 percent. Women exhibiting symptoms were more likely to transmit the virus. Lallemant further noted that three children who were HIV-1-negative at 12 and 15 months later became HIV-infected and concluded that breastfeeding was the most probable route of infection.

Becquart (1998) reported that 22/43 (52 percent) of children breastfed by HIV-1-infected mothers in Bangui, Central African Republic, became infected. Because stopping breastfeeding at age 6 months did not substan-tially reduce the risk of transmission, HIV-infected mothers may be better advised to breastfeed for a shorter time or not at all.

Leroy and colleagues (1998) in their multicenter pooled analysis of other studies about late postnatal transmission of HIV to breastfeeding children, concluded that the cumulative additional risk of infection was 2.5 percent at 12 months, 6.3 percent at 18 months, 7.4 percent at 24 months and 9.2 per-cent at 36 months. Thus ceasing breastfeeding after four to six months would spare some children. Breastfeeding after this time is not balanced with a com-parable reduction in non-HIV-related mortality.

## Infection During Birth Not Distinguishable From Infection Shortly After Birth

Although PCR results can determine in the early weeks if a baby is HIV-infected, PCRs cannot distinguish between infection acquired during birth from infection acquired shortly thereafter. PCR tests can tell only approximately when HIV infection takes place, but not exactly when, and not by what means. CDC's Bertolli and colleagues (1996) reported that for 261 HIV-1-infected mothers in Zaire, the overall rate of transmission was 26 percent. PCRs indicated that transmission in utero happened in 23 percent of cases. Transmission during delivery and the early postpartum period occurred in 65 percent of the cases. Late transmission (after 3–5 months) occurred in 12 percent of the cases.

Bertolli and colleagues noted that, even with PCR results, it was still not possible to distinguish between children who were infected during birth from those who became infected shortly thereafter through breastfeeding. They stated that their inability to distinguish between intrapartum and early postpartum transmission through breastfeeding may have led them to underestimate the frequency with which the latter occurred.

Simonon and colleagues (1994) in Rwanda also used PCR testing to follow children breastfed by HIV-1-positive mothers. Children were breastfed for a median of 579 days, with the duration of breastfeeding ranging from 0 to 1302 days. These researchers also noted the difficulties in distinguishing between means of transmission. They estimated that postnatal transmission via breastfeeding might be responsible for one- to two-thirds of mother-to-child HIV infections.

Ekpini and colleagues (1997) reported late postnatal mother-to-child transmission among children breastfed by HIV-positive women in Abidjan, Côte d'Ivoire. They used PCR testing to study children born to 138 HIV-1-positive mothers, 132 HIV-2-positive women, 69 women who were positive for both HIV-1 and HIV-2, and 274 HIV-negative women. They made diagnoses of late transmission if a child was negative by PCR at 3 or 6 months of age and then was positive by PCR at 9 months of age or persistently positive at age 15 months or older. They found that 28 percent of the babies of HIV-1-infected mothers became infected by 6 months of age, compared to 18 percent of babies born to mothers who were infected with both HIV-1 and HIV-2. They noted that 12 percent of breastfed children who escaped HIV-1 in the first six months became HIV-1-infected later. Among children who were breastfed by HIV-1-positive mothers until age 24 months, 20 percent acquired infection by that age. The researchers noted that the true rate of postnatal transmission may even exceed their estimates, since some children who tested HIV-positive by PCR after 6 months of life may have acquired their infection through breastmilk.

Guay and colleagues (1996) reported that 26.2 percent of children breastfed by 201 HIV-1-positive women in Uganda became HIV-1-positive. The researchers used PCR to look for the presence of HIV-1 in breastmilk and followed the children for at least two years. They found no correlation between either the detection of HIV-1 in breastmilk or the duration of breastfeeding and the risk of transmission. Mothers who transmitted HIV averaged 15.8 months of breastfeeding, which was not significantly different from the duration of 14.4 months for mothers who did not transmit.

Waloch (1997) reported very high rates of HIV transmission resulting from prolonged breastfeeding by 113 Zambian mothers, many of whom were symptomatic. The overall mother-to-child transmission rate was 90 percent. The mothers with most advanced HIV disease transmitted HIV to their babies in 94.7 percent of the cases.

## Prolonged Breastfeeding Outside of Africa

Al-Nozha and colleagues (1995) in Saudi Arabia reported the cases of nine children who had been HIV-1-infected by their mothers. The women had been infected either by blood transfusions before pregnancy or by sexual contact with husbands who had been transfusion-infected. By age 16 months, all nine children born to HIV-1-infected mothers were infected. As no PCR or virus culture tests were performed in the early weeks, it is impossible to know whether these nine children were infected in utero, during birth or by breastfeeding. Breastfeeding up to 2 years of age is common in Saudi Arabia.

Kumar and colleagues (1995) reported the results from a study in India of 143 HIV-1-positive mothers, 137 of whom were symptomatic. In all cases, it was believed that the women had been HIV-1-infected through heterosexual contact. The rate of transmission was 48 percent. It is not known how many babies were infected in utero, how many during birth or how many via breastfeeding. The authors noted that 74/143 children were born to and breastfed by HIV-1-positive mothers without becoming infected.

## Factors That Increase or Decrease Risk of Transmission

That all infected breastfeeding mothers do not transmit HIV-1 to their infants suggests the presence of factors either in the mother, the breastmilk or the child that prevent transmission. Some researchers have looked beyond the known factors that increase risk of transmission (such as longer duration of breastfeeding and higher maternal viral loads). Orloff (1993) suggested that a factor in human milk can sometimes inactivate HIV-1 and that this may explain why all babies breastfed by HIV-infected mothers do not become infected. Newburg and colleagues (1995) used the term "glycosaminoglycan" to describe a specific carbohydrate-containing molecule that can protect some babies from becoming HIV-infected through breastmilk.

Maternal factors that increase risk of transmission include a primary

infection during breastfeeding, symptomatic HIV disease, maternal immunosupression, high concentration of cell-free or cell-associated HIV in breastmilk, poor nutritional state (especially vitamin A deficiency), vaginal delivery especially with prolonged rupture of membranes, presence of maternal
breast/nipple problems, and long-term breastfeeding.

Factors in the child that increase the risk of infection include prematu-
rity, compromised mucosal barrier through inflammation or ulcers (of the
mouth, throat, esophagus, stomach, and intestines), thrush, teething, and gastroenteritis. With so many variables, it is understandable that the rates of
transmission vary greatly. But among children breastfed for at least three
months, rates of transmission are fairly high.

## Rates of Transmission Among Children
## Breastfed for Three Months or Longer

| Rate | Country | Researcher | Year |
|------|---------|------------|------|
| 25% | Rwanda | Simonon | 1994 |
| 26% | Uganda | Guay | 1996 |
| 26% | Zaire | Bertolli | 1996 |
| 30% | Brazil | Tess | 1997 |
| 30% | Tanzania | Karlsson | 1997 |
| 39% | Zaire | Ryder | 1989 |
| 35% | Malawi | Taha | 1995 |
| 35% | Soweto | Gray | 1997 |
| 38% | South Africa | Bobat | 1997 |
| 40% | Congo | Lallemant | 1994 |
| 43% | Kenya | Datta | 1994 |
| 48% | India | Kumar | 1995 |
| 49% | Brazil | Rubini | 1996 |
| 52% | Central African Republic | Becquart | 1998 |
| 57% | Spain | Maguire | 1997 |
| 63% | Italy | Gabiano | 1992 |
| 90% | Zambia | Waloch | 1997 |

# References

Adams, D. S., et al. 1984. Global survey of evidence of capine arthritis-encephalitis virus infection. *Veterinary Research* 115: 493–495.

*Affordable Options for the Prevention of Mother-to-Child Transmission of HIV-1.* 1997. Johannesburg, South Africa, November 19–20. National AIDS Programme and the Perinatal HIV Research Unit.

Al-Nozha, M. M., A. R. Al-Frath, M. Al-Nasser and S. Ramia. 1995. Horizontal versus vertical transmission of human immunodeficiency virus type 1 (HIV-1). *Tropical and Geographical Medicine* 47(6): 293–295.

Avila, M. M., et al. 1997. HIV-1 transmission through breast-feeding in Argentina. Presented at the Conference on Global Strategies for the Prevention of HIV Transmission from Mothers to Infants, Washington, D.C. September 3–6.

Becquart, P., et al. 1998. Early postnatal mother-to-child transmission of HIV-1 in Bangui, Central African Republic. Presented at the Fifth Conference on Retroviruses and Opportunistic Infections, Chicago, Illinois, February 1–5.

Bélec, Laurent, et al. 1990. Antibodies to human immunodeficiency virus in the breast milk of healthy, seropositive women. *Pediatrics* 85: 1022–1026.

Bertolli, Jeanne, et al. 1996. Estimating the timing of mother-to-child transmission of human immunodeficiency virus in a breast-feeding population in Kinshasa, Zaire. *Journal of Infectious Diseases* 174: 722–726.

Black, Rebecca F. 1996. Transmission of HIV-1 in the breast-feeding process. *Journal of the American Dietetic Association* 96: 267–274.

Blanche, S., et al. 1989. A prospective study of perinatal infection of infants born to women seropositive for human immunodeficiency virus type 1. *New England Journal of Medicine* 320: 1643–1648.

Bobat, R., Moodley Dhayendree, Anna Coutsoudis and Hoosen Coovadia. 1997. Breastfeeding by HIV-1-infected women and outcome in their infants: A cohort study from Durban, South Africa. *AIDS* 11: 1627–1633.

Bulterys, M., A. Chao, A. Dushimimana and A. Saah. 1995. HIV-1 seroconversion after 20 months in a cohort of breastfed children born to HIV-1-infected women in Rwanda. *AIDS* 9(1): 93–94.

Caterino-De-Araulo, Adele, and E. Santos-Fortuna. 1998. No evidence of vertical transmission of HTLV-I and HTLV-II in children at high risk of HIV-1 infection from São Paulo, Brazil. Presented at the Twelfth World AIDS Conference, Geneva, Switzerland, June 28–July 3. Abstract 23307.

Centers for Disease Control and Prevention, USPHS Working Group. 1993. Guidelines for counseling persons infected with human T-lymphotrophic virus type I (HTLV-I) and type II (HTLV-II). *Annals of Internal Medicine* 118: 448–454.

Colebunders, Robert, et al. 1988. Breast-feeding and transmission of HIV. *Lancet* ii: 1487.

Daar, E. S., R. D. Moudgil, R. D. Meyer and D. D. Ho. 1991. Transient high levels of viremia in patients with primary human immunodeficiency virus type 1 infection. *New England Journal of Medicine* 334: 961–964.

Dabis, François, et al. 1992. Estimating the rate of mother-to-child transmission of HIV. Report of a workshop on methodological issues, Ghent, Belgium, 17–22 February 1992. *AIDS* 7: 1139–1148.

Datta, Pratibha, Joanne E. Embree and Joan K. Kreiss. 1992. Resumption of breast-feeding in later childhood: A risk factor for mother-to-child human immunodeficiency virus type 1 transmission. *Pediatric Infectious Disease Journal* 11: 974–976.

Datta, Pratibha, et al. 1994. Mother-to-child transmission of human immunodeficiency virus type 1: Report from the Nairobi study. *Journal of Infectious Diseases* 170: 1134–1140.

De Cock, Kevin M., et al. 1994. Retrospective study of maternal HIV-1 and HIV-2 infections and child survival in Abidjan, Côte d'Ivoire. *British Medical Journal* 308 (6925): 441–443.

De Martino, Maurizio, et al. 1992. HIV-1 transmission through breast milk: Appraisal of the risk according to duration of feeding. *AIDS* 6: 991–997.

De Martino, M., and Pier-Angelo Tovo. 1993. Quantifying the risk of HIV-1 transmission via breast-milk (reply). *AIDS* 7: 134–135.

De Martino, M., et al. 1994a. Features of children perinatally infected with HIV-1 surviving longer than 5 years. *Lancet* 343: 191–195.

_____, et al. 1994b. Human immunodeficiency virus type 1 infection and breast milk. *Acta Paediatrica Supplement* 400: 51–58.

Duprat, Christine, et al. 1994. Human immunodeficiency virus type 1 IgA antibody in breast milk and serum. *Pediatric Infectious Disease Journal* 13: 603–608.

Ekpini, E., S. Z. Wiktor and T. Sibailly. 1994. Late postnatal mother-to-child HIV transmission in Abidjan, Côte d'Ivoire. Presented at the Tenth International Conference on AIDS, Yokohama, Japan, August. Abstract 218C.

Ekpini, Ehounou R., et al. 1997. Late postnatal mother-to-child transmission of HIV-1 in Abidjan, Côte d'Ivoire. *Lancet* 349: 1054–1059.

Flores, Guerrero. 1991. Postnatal transmission of the human immunodeficiency virus (HIV). History of brief breast-feeding. *Ginecologa Obstetrica of Mexico* 59: 117–121.

Frederick, Toni, et al. 1997. Breastfeeding and disease progression among perinatally HIV-infected children in Los Angeles. Presented at the Fourth Conference on Retroviruses and Opportunistic Infections, Washington, D.C., January 22–27. Abstract 733.

Frenkel, Lisa M., et al. 1998. Genetic evaluation of suspected cases of transient HIV-1 infection of infants. *Science* 280: 1073.

Gabiano, C., et al. 1991. HIV-1 transmission rate in first-born children to seropositive mothers and interfering factors. Presented at the Seventh International Conference on AIDS, Florence, Italy, June 16–21.

Global Programme on AIDS. 1992. Consensus statement from the WHO/UNICEF Constitution on HIV transmission and breast feeding. *Weekly Epidemiological Record* 67: 177–184.

Gray, Glenda E. 1997. Breastfeeding-related transmission. Presented at the Fourth International Conference on AIDS in Asia and the Pacific, Manila, Philippines, October 25–29. Abstract FA10.

Guay, Laura, et al. 1996. Detection of human immunodeficiency virus type 1

(HIV-1) DNA and p24 antigen in breast milk of HIV-1-infected Ugandan women and vertical transmission. *Pediatrics* 98: 438–444.

Heneine, W., et al. 1992. Detection of HTLV-II in breast milk of HTLV-II infected mothers (Letter). *Lancet* 340: 1157–1158.

Hino, S., et al. 1985. Mother-to-child transmission of human T-cell leukemia virus type-1. *Japanese Cancer Research* 76: 474–480.

Hira, S. K., et al. 1989. Perinatal transmission of HIV-1 in Zambia. *British Medical Journal* 299: 1250–1252.

Hira, S. K., et al. 1990. Apparent vertical transmission of human immunodeficiency virus type 1 by breast-feeding in Zambia. *Journal of Pediatrics* 117 (3): 421–424.

Hoover, Kay. 1997. Candidiasis and breastfeeding. Presented at the 1997 International Conference on the Theory and Practice of Human Lactation, Orlando, Florida, January 16–19.

Kaplan, Jonathan E., et al. 1992. Low risk of mother-to-child transmission of human T-lymphotropic virus type II in non-breast-fed infants. *Journal of Infectious Diseases* 166: 892–895.

Karlsson, Katrina, et al. 1997. Late postnatal transmission of human immunodeficiency virus type 1 infection from mothers to infants in Dar es Salaam, Tanzania. *Pediatric Infectious Disease Journal* 16: 963–967.

Kawase, Ken-ichiro, et al. 1992. Maternal transmission of HTLV-1 other than through breast milk: Discrepancy between the polymerase china reaction positivity of cord blood samples for HTLV-1 and the subsequent seropositivity of individuals. *Japanese Journal of Cancer Research* 83: 968–977.

Krivine, A., S. Le Bourdelles, G. Firtion and P. Lebon. 1997. Viral kinetics in HIV-1 perinatal infection. *Lancet* 350: 493.

Kreiss, J. 1997. Breastfeeding and vertical transmission of HIV-1. *Acta Paediatrica Supplement* 421: 113–117.

Kumar, Rachana M., Sayenna A. Uduman and Ashok K. Khurranna. 1995. A prospective study of mother-to-infant HIV transmission in tribal women from India. *Journal of Acquired Immune Deficiency Syndromes* 9: 238–242.

Lallemant, Marc, et al. 1994a. Mother-to-child transmission of HIV-1 in Congo, Central African Republic. *AIDS* 8: 1451–1456.

Lallemant, M., S. Le Coeur, D. Tarantola, J. Mann and M. Essex. 1994b. Preventing perinatal transmission. *Lancet* 343: 1429–1430.

Lepage, Philippe, et al. 1987. Postnatal transmission of HIV from mother to child. *Lancet* ii: 400.

Leroy, Valeriane, et al. 1998. Late postnatal mother-to-child transmission (LPT) of HIV-1: International muticentre pooled analysis. In *Mother-to-Child HIV Transmission: New Findings*. Proceedings of the Twelfth World Conference on AIDS, Geneva, Switzerland, July 1.

Lewis, Paul, et al. 1998. Cell-free human immunodeficiency virus type 1 in breast milk. *Journal of Infectious Diseases* 177: 34–39.

Lyons, Susan F., et al. 1996. Mother-to-infant transmission of HIV-1 in South Africa. Presented at the Eleventh International Conference on AIDS, Vancouver, Canada, July 7–12. Abstract Tu.C.2579.

Maguire, A., et al. 1997. Potential risk factors for vertical HIV-1 transmission in Catalonia, Spain: The protective role of Cesarean section. *AIDS* 11: 1851–1857.

Macdonald, Kelly S., et al. 1998. Class I MHC polymorphism and mother-to-child HIV-1 transmission in Kenya. In *Mother-to-Child HIV Transmission: Biological Determinants.* Proceedings of the Twelfth World AIDS Conference, Geneva, Switzerland, June 30.

Malaviya, A. N., et al. 1992. Circumstantial evidence of HIV transmission via breast milk. *Journal of Acquired Immune Deficiency Syndromes* 5: 102–106.

Marlink, R., et al. 1997. Lessons from the second AIDS virus, HIV-2. Presented at the National Conference on HIV/AIDS, Gaborone, Botswana, August 6–9.

McDonald, A., et al. 1996. Perinatal exposure to HIV in Australia, 1982–1995. Presented at the Annual Conference by Australia's Society for HIV Medicine, Sydney, Australia, November 14–17.

Miotti, Paolo G., et al. 1996. Additional HIV infection in children born to HIV-infected women and not infected at birth or in the first weeks of life. Presented at the Eleventh International Conference on AIDS, Vancouver, Canada, July 7–12. Abstract Tu.C.2605.

Mussi-Pinhata, Marisa M., et. al. 1998. Congenital and perinatal cytomegalovirus infection in infants born to mothers infected with human immunodeficiency virus. *Journal of Pediatrics* 132: 285–290.

Nagelkerke, Nico J. D., et al. 1995. The duration of breastfeeding by HIV-infected mothers in resource-poor countries: Balancing benefits and risks. *Journal of Acquired Immune Deficiency Syndromes* 8: 176–181.

Nduati, Ruth W., Grace C. John and J. Kreiss. 1994. Postnatal transmission of HIV-1 through pooled breast milk. *Lancet* 344: 1432.

Nduati, Ruth W., Grace C. John and Barbra A. Richardson. 1995. Human immunodeficiency virus type 1-infected cells in breast milk: Association with immunosupression and vitamin A deficiency. *Journal of Infectious Diseases* 172: 1461–1468.

Newburg, David S., Robert J. Linhardt, Stephen A. Ampofo and Robert H. Yolken. 1995. Human milk glycosaminoglycans inhibit HIV glycoprotein gp 120 binding to its host cell CD4 receptor. *Journal of Nutrition* 125: 419–424.

Nicoll, Angus, et al. 1995. Infant feeding policy and practice in the presence of HIV-1 infection. *AIDS* 9: 107–119.

Njenga, Simon, et al. 1997. Risk factors for postnatal mother-to-child transmission of HIV-1 in Nairobi. Presented at the Conference on Global Strategies for the Prevention of HIV Transmission from Mothers to Infants, Washington, D.C., September 3–6.

O'Donovan, Diarmuid, et al. 1997. A community-based study of perinatal and postnatal transmission of HIV-1 and HIV-2 in The Gambia, West Africa. Presented at the Conference on Global Strategies for the Prevention of HIV Transmission from Mothers to Infants, Washington, D.C., September 3–6.

Opperman, Edith. 1997. To breast-feed or not to breast-feed: That is the question in Zimbabwe. Presented at the Conference on Global Strategies for the Prevention of HIV Transmission from Mothers to Infants, Washington, D.C., September 3–6.

Orloff, S. L., et al. 1993. Inactivation of human immunodeficiency virus type 1 in human milk: Effects of intrinsic factors in human milk and of pasteurization. *Journal of Human Lactation* 9: 13–17.

Ota, Martin, et al. 1998. Influence of maternal HIV-1 and HIV-2 on child survival in The Gambia. In *Mother-to-Child HIV Transmission: Biological Determinants.* Proceedings of the Twelfth World AIDS Conference, Geneva, Switzerland, June 30.

Palasanthiran, P., et al. 1993. Breast-feeding during primary maternal human immunodeficiency virus infection and risk of transmission from mother to infant. *Journal of Infectious Diseases* 167: 141–444.

Ravinathan, Ramanathan, et al. 1996. Prevention of mother-to-child transmission through perinatal care. Presented at the Eleventh International Conference on AIDS, Vancouver, Canada, July 7–12. Abstract We.C.3580.

Rubini, Norma de Paula Motta, and Leigh J. Passman. 1992. Transmission of human immunodeficiency virus infection from a newly infected mother to her two-year-old child by breastfeeding. *Pediatric Infectious Disease Journal* 11: 682–683.

Rubini, Norma de Paula Motta, et al. 1996. HIV vertical transmission in Rio de Janeiro: Rate and risk factors. Presented at the Eleventh International Conference on AIDS, Vancouver, Canada, July 7–12. Abstract Tu.C. 2570.

Ruff, A. J., et al. 1994. Prevalence of HIV-1 DNA and p24 antigen in breast milk and correlation with maternal factors. *Journal of Acquired Immune Deficiency Syndromes* 7: 68–73.

Simonon, Arlette, et al. 1994. An assessment of the timing of mother-to-child transmission of human immunodeficiency virus type 1 by means of polymerase chain reaction. *Journal of Acquired Immune Deficiency Syndromes* 7: 952–957.

Stiehm, E. Richard, and Peter Vink. 1991. Transmission of human immunodeficiency virus infection by breast-feeding. *Journal of Pediatrics* 118 (3): 410–412.

Taha, Taha E., et al. 1995. The effect of human immunodeficiency virus infection on birthweight, infant and child mortality in urban Malawi. *International Journal of Epidemiology* 24(5): 1022–1029.

_____. 1998. HIV infection due to breastfeeding in a cohort of babies not infected at enrollment. Presented at the Twelfth World AIDS Conference, Geneva, Switzerland, June 30–July 3. Abstract 23270.

Tarantola, Daniel J. M., and Jonathan M. Mann, eds. 1996. *AIDS in the World II.* New York: Oxford University Press.

Tess, Beatriz H., et al. 1998. Breastfeeding, genetic, obstetric and other risk factors associated with mother-to-child transmission of HIV-1 in São Paulo State, Brazil. *AIDS* 12: 513–520.

Thiry, L., et al. 1985. Isolation of AIDS virus from cell-free breast milk of three healthy virus carriers. *Lancet* ii: 891–892.

Tovo, Pier-Angelo, et al. 1994. AIDS appearance in children is associated with the velocity of disease progression in their mothers. *Journal of Infectious Diseases* 170: 1000–1002.

Tozzi, A. E., et al. 1990. Does breast-feeding delay progression to AIDS in HIV-infected children? (Letter). *AIDS* 4: 1293–1294.

Travers, K. U., et al. 1998. Protection from HIV-1 infection by HIV-2. *AIDS* 12: 222–223.

UNAIDS Joint United Nations Programme on HIV/AIDS. 1996. HIV and Infant Feeding: An Interim Statement. *Weekly Epidemiological Record* 71: 289–291.

_____. 1997a. *Breastfeeding and HIV/AIDS*. Geneva, Switzerland: UNAIDS.

_____. 1997b. *HIV and Infant Feeding*. A Policy Statement. Geneva, Switzerland: UNAIDS.

_____. 1997c. *Report on the Global HIV/AIDS Epidemic*. Geneva, Switzerland: UNAIDS.

Van de Perre, Philippe, Deo-Gratis Hitimana and Philippe Lepage. 1988. Human immunodeficiency virus antibodies of IgG, IgA, and IgM subclasses in milk of seropositive mothers. *Journal of Pediatrics* 113 (6): 1039–1041.

Van de Perre, Philippe, et al. 1991. Postnatal transmission of human immunodeficiency virus type 1 from mother to infant. A prospective cohort study in Kigali, Rwanda. *New England Journal of Medicine* 325: 593–598.

_____, et al. 1992. Postnatal transmission of HIV-1 associated with breast abscess (Letter). *Lancet* 339: 1490–1491.

_____, et al. 1993. Infective and anti-infective properties of breastmilk from HIV-1-infected women. *Lancet* 341: 914–918.

Van de Perre, P. 1995. Epidemiology of HIV infection & AIDS in Africa. *Trends Microbiology* 3: 217–222.

Vochem, Matthias, Klaus Hamprecht, Gerhard Jahn and Christian P. Speer. 1998. Transmission of cytomegalovirus to preterm infants through breast milk. *Pediatric Infectious Disease Journal* 17: 53–58.

Waloch, Marek, C. M. Njovu, P. C. Chanda and M. Kabole. 1997 Retrospective and prospective study of children born to HIV symptomatic mothers and consequences. Presented at the Conference on Global Strategies for the Prevention of HIV Transmission from Mothers to Infants, Washington, D.C., September 3–6.

Weinbreck, P., et al. 1988. Postnatal transmission of HIV infection. *Lancet* i: 482.

World Health Organization. 1987. Breast-feeding/breast milk and human immunodeficiency virus (HIV). *Weekly Epidemiological Record* 33: 245–246.

Ziegler, John B., David A. Cooper, Richard O. Johnson and Julian Gold. 1985. Postnatal transmission of AIDS-associated retrovirus from mother to infant. *Lancet* ii: 896–897.

# CHAPTER THREE

# Other Issues
# in Mother-to-Child
# HIV Transmission

If HIV-infected mothers avoid breastfeeding, they can reduce the risk of infecting their babies by approximately one-half. But since it is not possible to distinguish babies infected during birth from babies infected by breastfeeding shortly thereafter, one also needs to take into account research about transmission during delivery. When mothers are given antiretroviral drugs such as AZT before and during birth, their babies are significantly less likely to become HIV-infected at that time. But the more babies are protected through birth, the greater the proportion of babies who will become infected through breastfeeding. Another reason discussions about drugs such as AZT relate to breastfeeding is the suggestion that babies or mothers may be placed on such drugs during breastfeeding.

## A Package of Interventions

Based on research available through mid–1998, one can list various inventions that definitely or possibly affect the risk of mother-to-child transmission. Treating mothers with antiretroviral drugs such as AZT and avoiding breastfeeding clearly reduce risk. Many studies suggest that performing cesarean deliveries reduce the risk of HIV transmission (European Collaborative Study 1994 and 1996, Kuhn 1996, Peckham and Newell 1997, Mandelbrot 1998). Cesareans performed before women go into labor were more protective than those performed during labor (Shaffer 1998). French researchers found that cesareans protected only babies of women who were treated with AZT (Mandelbrot 1998). The reduced transmission risk associated with cesareans, however, must be balanced against the procedure-related complications and the mother's increased mortality rate. In developing countries, HIV-positive women who had cesarean deliveries had a much higher mortality rate than comparable women who had vaginal deliveries (Bulterys 1996).

Minimizing the baby's exposure to the mother's blood and body fluids also appears to be protective. When women in labor rupture membranes—when their "water breaks"—for more than four hours before delivery, their babies are more likely to be infected (Landesman 1996, Kuhn 1997). Results of research now in progress will indicate how effective it is to give women vitamin A supplements or perform vaginal cleansing during labor and delivery.

The use of antiretroviral drugs is an extremely important part of a package of interventions. In the mid–1990s, attention to the topic of mother-to-child HIV transmission focused primarily not on breastfeeding, but on the use of drugs. In August 1997, it was announced that there were 37 clinical trials studying mother-to-child transmission (Fowler 1997). Of these 37, 21 studies involve antiretroviral drugs, while only one involves breast versus formula feeding. This study is being conducted in Nairobi, Kenya, with 409 HIV-positive women who have been randomly assigned to breast or formula-feed.

## Antiretroviral Drug Therapy

The use of antiretroviral drugs, which attack retroviruses like HIV-1 and HIV-2, has been the biggest success story in the field of HIV/AIDS, and drug therapy has become a major focus of discussion about mother-to-child HIV transmission. AZT (or zidovudine) has long been the best-known antiretroviral drug. AZT, 3TC, ddI, ddc, d4T and abacavir belong to the category of antiretroviral drugs called nucleoside reverse transcriptase inhibitors. They work by blocking the function of a crucial enzyme (reverse transcriptase), thereby disrupting an early stage in the replication of the virus. Nevirapine and delavirdine are examples of nonnucleoside reverse transcriptase inhibitors. They directly inactivate the same enzyme, reverse transcriptase. The protease inhibitors, such as ritonavir, indinavir, nelfinavir and saquinavir, work at a later stage to stop new virus copies from infecting other cells.

Antiretroviral drugs slow the progression to symptomatic HIV disease (AIDS). Most people who take the drugs feel better and improve in their laboratory test results (raised CD4 counts and reduced viral loads). Some HIV-1-infected persons in wealthy industrialized countries are now offered the option of receiving early, aggressive treatment with triple-drug combinations. The idea of drug therapy is to hit the virus hard and early with highly active anti-retroviral therapy (HAART). The potent combination of antiretroviral drugs can often reduce the virus level in the bloodstream to undetectable levels. Drug therapies, however, do not "cure" people of AIDS. The virus instead "hides" in resting immune system cells (Chun 1997). There is a residual pool of HIV even after prolonged combination therapy (Ho 1998). Combination drug therapy has, nevertheless, made great progress in improving the quality and duration of life for the relatively few people who can afford it or who qualify for limited governmental or drug company support.

Dr. Peter Piot, executive director of UNAIDS, noted another problem with combination therapy: Its success has made people complacent about AIDS. Such unconcern is unlikely to stop the rapid spread of HIV/AIDS or to extend care to people in resource-poor nations (Piot 1997). In addition to the major problems of price, availability and complacency, there are other problems with antiretoviral drug therapy, including serious side effects, complicated dosing schedules and concerns about drug resistance or rebounding viral levels after discontinuing drug therapy.

## *ACTG 076: A Reduction Greater Than What Is Expected from Vaccines*

In 1994 Connor and colleagues announced an extremely important study. The Pediatric AIDS Clinical Trials Group Protocol (ACTG 076) was conducted by researchers in France and the United States. The study indicated that giving the drug AZT to pregnant women and giving it to the baby for the first six weeks cut the chance of transmitting HIV-1 to the baby by 67 percent (Connor 1994). In the group in which the mother-baby pairs received the AZT, the risk of transmission was only 8.3 percent, as compared to a rate of 25.5 percent for the group that received the placebo. All babies were formula-fed.

The results of ACTG 076 revolutionized the recommended treatment of pregnant HIV-positive women. Pizzo and Wilfert (1995) referred to the study as the "most stunning and important result in clinical acquired immuno-deficiency syndrome research to date." Dr. Arthur Ammann, Chairman of the American Foundation for AIDS Research, noted that even the most optimistic predictions place eventual vaccine efficacy at around 50 percent protection, compared to the 60–70 percent reduction with perinatal AZT (Ammann 1997).

## *Steps Beyond ACTG 076 in Affluent Countries*

Kind and colleagues in Switzerland (1998) reported the effectiveness of various interventions. Thirty-one women received AZT plus elective cesarean delivery; their rate of transmission was zero. Eighty-six women received elective cesarean delivery, but no AZT; their rate of transmission was 8 percent (7/86 babies were HIV-infected). Twenty-four women received AZT alone and no cesarean; their rate of transmission was 17 percent (4/24 babies were HIV-infected). Cesareans, then, in this group of women, were more effective than antiretroviral drug therapy. The researchers also reported that 271 women had received no treatment in previous years; their rate of transmission was 20 percent (55/271 babies were HIV-infected). Among 133 HIV-positive French women who were treated with AZT and delivered via a planned cesarean, only one baby became infected (Mandelbrot 1998).

In 1997 the United States Public Health Service issued new recommendations for the use of antiretroviral drugs with HIV-1-infected pregnant women in the United States (Office of Public Health 1997). The report noted that antiretroviral monotherapy (one-drug therapy) is now considered suboptimal for the treatment of HIV-1-infection in general. Since AZT alone is suboptimal for nonpregnant individuals, it is also suboptimal for pregnant individuals. Pregnant HIV-1-infected women, to best control their own HIV disease, should be treated as if they were not pregnant. Pregnant women, however, may want to consider not taking antiretroviral drugs in the first 10–12 weeks of pregnancy. The children of women who took AZT in pregnancy had no higher risk of birth defects or other problems, but further monitoring will be needed to rule out possible adverse effects on the developing fetus. Pregnant women should be fully informed of all options.

Although AZT monotherapy has been proven effective in preventing mother-to-child transmission, it has disadvantages. Monotherapy, for instance, is not as effective as combination therapies in controlling the HIV disease of the mother. Furthermore, monotherapy can increase the odds of drug resistance, which may later reduce the treatment options for both the mother and the child who was exposed to AZT as a fetus.

Beyond questions of efficacy, there is the concern that, for most of the world, monotherapy with AZT is too expensive. In many resource-poor countries, the national health budget is often less than U.S.$10 per person per year. The stark contrast between how much health care is available in industrialized countries and how little is available in resource-poor countries is exemplified by recent medical journal articles. While Kind (1998) reported a zero percent transmission rate with AZT and cesareans in Switzerland, Waloch and colleagues (1997) reported a 90 percent transmission rate among symptomatic Zambian women. One could retort that other studies show only a 26–52 percent transmission rate with prolonged breastfeeding, and that the 90 percent rate in Zambia was due to the fact that the women were symptomatic. But, then again, their symptomatic status is related to the fact that they were in Zambia. If they were in an industrialized country, they would likely have received antiretroviral drugs and would be much less symptomatic or even asymptomatic. Much of it comes down to the stark differences between the financial resources of the countries. Zambia does not have the financial resources to routinely provide AZT, counseling and testing programs, or cesarean deliveries or even safe alternatives to breastfeeding.

## Trials That Followed ACTG 076

The 1994 announcement of the success of ACTG 076 led to many other clinical trials of drug therapies for pregnant HIV-positive women. In ACTG 076, AZT monotherapy was delivered in a specific dosing regimen for the last sixteen to twenty-four weeks of pregnancy, plus intravenous administration during labor, and dosing newborns for six weeks after birth. There was no breastfeeding.

The regimen in ACTG 076 became the standard of care in countries that could afford AZT, and was also used with HIV-infected women in some less developed countries. Indeed, the results in the Bahama Islands were very similar to the results in the original ACTG 076. The AZT monotherapy reduced mother-to-child transmission to 7.4 percent, compared to the 28 percent transmission rate that had been found previously (Gomez 1997). The Bahamian babies were not breastfed.

Researchers in India reported good results with AZT plus chlorhexidine douches used hourly during labor (Staple 1997). Thirty-eight HIV-positive women (asymptomatic or with CD4 counts greater than 200) completed the therapy that used oral AZT. The drug was administered in the third trimester of pregnancy, during labor and for the first six weeks postpartum for both mother and baby. Of these 38 babies, only six (15.8 percent) became HIV-infected. The Indian babies were not breastfed.

One of the international trials designed to test the effectiveness of an intervention that is cheaper and simpler than ACTG 076 has been conducted in Thailand and in Côte d'Ivoire by researchers from the two countries and the United States. In February 1998 the Thai and U.S. researchers announced a great success (Joint Statement 1998). Short-term use of AZT had lowered the risk of perinatal transmission by 51 percent (from 18.6 percent without AZT to 9.2 percent with AZT). Principal researcher Dr. Nathan Shaffer announced this was the first time that there was conclusive scientific proof that AZT, given late in pregnancy, really works to reduce HIV transmission. The 19-month study had involved 397 HIV-positive Thai women, who were given AZT orally twice daily beginning at 36 weeks of pregnancy. During labor AZT was administered every three hours. The Thai babies were all formula-fed, so none risked subsequent HIV infection.

At the Côte d'Ivoire site, pregnant HIV-positive women are being treated with oral AZT, but then breastfeed. The results of this study will go far in quantifying the additional risk associated with breastfeeding by women previously treated with AZT.

Shortly after the Thai results were announced, UNAIDS convened a meeting in Geneva. Glaxo Wellcome, the manufacturer of AZT, agreed to reduce the price of the drug by as much as 75 percent for pregnant HIV-positive women in resource-poor countries. The price cut is intended only to decrease mother-to-child transmission, and will not provide long-term treatment to mothers (Waldholz 1998).

Those in attendance at the UNAIDS meeting called for concerted international action in preventing mother-to-child transmission of HIV. They emphasized this must become a global health priority. Dr. Piot of UNAIDS echoed the concern of participants that delay could only lead to a significant deterioration in the situation (UNAIDS 1998). The UNAIDS position was that HIV-positive women should be advised not to breastfeed, and making antiretroviral drugs, HIV tests and breastmilk substitutes affordable and available should be an important priority.

## Other Trials of Antiretroviral Drugs

In addition to their studies of AZT monotherapy, researchers are investigating the merits of other singly administered reverse transcriptase inhibitors and the efficacy of combination therapy. Scientists have found, for instance, that AZT works well in combination with the drug 3TC. The drug nevirapine (a non-nucleoside reverse transcriptase inhibitor) has the disadvantage that people quickly become resistant to it, but is considered an excellent candidate for reducing transmission during birth. It is readily absorbed, with high blood levels reached in two hours. The high levels are immediately transferred to the baby. Researchers have found that the babies at birth had levels equal to the mothers' levels. They have seen no signs of nevirapine toxicity in mother or baby.

In industrialized countries, nevirapine is being tested against placebo, but in all cases the women also receive AZT and/or a similar drug. But in resource-poor countries, nevirapine is being tested alone. It is given in the form of one pill to the woman in labor and another pill to the newborn. The total cost is about U.S.$2.00. If this treatment proves to be as effective as is hoped, it could be widely used in resource-poor countries.

Dr. John Sullivan (1997) suggested that nevirapine treatment might even be used on a population-wide basis in a resource-poor country that does not have HIV testing generally available. If that were the case, *all* pregnant (untested) women in an endemic area would be treated with nevirapine. If the U.S.$2.00 nevirapine regimen is shown to be effective, it could be used in an area that does not have an HIV testing and counseling program.

Research into other alternatives to ACTG 076 is ongoing. A trial is being conducted of 1500 HIV-1-infected pregnant women in Uganda. It is designed to compare the effectiveness of a short course of oral AZT and a short course of oral nevirapine or placebo. The women will be treated once in labor, and the babies, who will be breastfed, will begin treatment after the first week.

The Perinatal Transmission Study (PETRA), which involves 1,960 HIV-1-infected women in five sites in Uganda, Tanzania and South Africa, is being conducted by UNAIDS. Subjects given a combination of AZT and 3TC in three different regimens will be monitored, with their condition compared at intervals to that of a control group. All sites were to have involved breastfeeding populations. The feeding plans, however, have changed. Many women in South Africa now choose to bottle-feed. And in Uganda and Tanzania, the breastfeeding recommendations were changed during a routine ethical review of the study. Originally, women would have breastfed for as long as they wanted. But researchers in these PETRA trials are now to advise women in Uganda and Tanzania to cease breastfeeding at six months postpartum. This newer recommendation was a response to research suggesting that long-term breastfeeding exposes babies to further risk of HIV infection without providing a comparable benefit.

Another trial is being conducted with 940 HIV-1-infected women in Ethiopia who receive one of two AZT regimens, with the prescription depending on whether mother and baby receive the drug after delivery. Babies are to be breastfed for three months.

An additional trial is being conducted at two sites, one in Côte d'Ivoire and the other in Burkina Faso, with 780 women. In one group AZT is given to the woman at the end of pregnancy, during labor and then for one week after delivery. The babies are not given AZT and are breastfed.

## A Heated Debate Over the International Trials

The use of placebos in the international trials became the focus of a heated debate in 1997 with coverage in daily newspapers. Critics argued that since AZT is known to reduce mother-to-child tranmission, it is unethical to offer a placebo. They reasoned that if it is unethical to use placebos with HIV-infected pregnant women in industrialized countries, it is unethical to offer placebos in other countries. Proponents of the trials argued that HIV-infected women in resource-poor countries would have received no treatment; therefore placebos do no harm. While providing antiretroviral drug treatment (free if necessary) to all pregnant women may be the standard of care in the United States, in resource-poor countries there is no such standard of care. They further argued that doing research with placebos is the fastest way to find answers. The sooner results are available, the sooner they can be applied to more mother-baby pairs.

Researchers from the CDC and from Côte d'Ivoire noted that while the debate focused on the ethics of using a placebo-controlled trial, other issues are of more immediate concern to them (Feinman 1997). They pointed out that the biggest issue is not the use of placebos, but whether the drug AZT will be made available to HIV-infected women in Africa. They also noted how difficult it is to recruit women into studies because women fear stigmatization and abandonment by their male partners.

## Affordable Interventions

There has been considerable interest in the use of micronutrients and vitamins, especially vitamin A, by pregnant or breastfeeding women. Interest in using vitamin A was sparked by reports that vitamin A–deficient women were significantly more likely to transmit HIV to their children than non–vitamin A–deficient women. Semba (1994) found, in a study in Malawi, that women with severe vitamin A deficiency had a transmission rate of 32.4 percent, compared to 7.2 percent for women with high vitamin A levels. In Kenya, Nduati and colleagues (1995) showed that vitamin A deficiency was correlated with an increased likelihood of women shedding virus in their milk if their HIV disease was advanced to the point of having CD4 counts below 400.

Vitamin A deficiency may result from dietary insufficiency, advanced HIV disease or both. Infection depletes vitamin A stores. Whether giving breastfeeding women extra vitamin A will make them less likely to transmit the virus in their milk is not yet known. What is known is that giving high doses of vitamin A supplements to breastfeeding mothers improves their vitamin A status, as well as their babies' (Stoltzfus 1993). In general, the quality of breastmilk remains remarkably high despite malnutrition; women, like other mammals, "milk off their backs" and give milk at the expense of their own bodies. But maternal vitamin A deficiency is one notable area where deficiency in the mother results in deficiency in breastmilk. Women who have been profoundly vitamin A deficient clearly have less vitamin A in their milk; this deficiency becomes worse as prolonged lactation continues in the face of maternal malnutrition.

In industrialized countries, where severe vitamin A deficiency is uncommon, however, breastfeeding women still transmitted HIV at high rates: 41 percent in Italy (Gabiano 1992), 57 percent in Spain (Maguire 1997), 83 percent in France (Blanche 1989) and 50 percent in Australia (McDonald 1996).

The ongoing international perinatal vitamin A trials will show whether giving vitamin A supplements protects babies during pregnancy, delivery or during breastfeeding. In these trials, some women will be given vitamin A and others placebo. Bell and colleagues (1997) argued that the cost and toxicity of vitamin A are so low, that it may be cost-effective and prudent to give vitamin A supplements routinely to all pregnant women. This action might prove worthwhile in an area where 12.5 percent of pregnant women are HIV-1-infected. Even if vitamin A supplements are shown not to significantly reduce the risk of mother-to-child transmission, they still provide other benefits.

Fawzi and colleagues (1998) reported that multivitamin supplementation substantially reduced adverse pregnancy outcomes (low birthweight, severely premature and small-for-gestational-age babies) and increased T-cell counts among HIV-positive women. Vitamin A supplements, however, did not significantly affect any of these outcomes. Whether supplements will decrease mother-to-child transmission or effect the clinical progression of HIV disease is not yet known.

Other relatively affordable interventions are aimed at reducing the baby's exposure to the mother's blood and secretions. To avoid opening a portal of entry, there should be no amniocentesis and no fetal monitoring with scalp electrodes. There should be no prolonged rupture of membranes, or no "breaking the water," to speed up labor and no routine episiotomies. Babies are to be wiped off. Whether routine suctioning of the baby's airways is beneficial or harmful is unknown. Suctioning can be harmful because it can scrape the baby's mouth or throat. Suctioning may prove beneficial because it removes maternal fluids.

Researchers had hoped that a simple cleansing of the birth canal of HIV-positive mothers during labor would reduce the risk of transmission. Vaginal cleansing can be done by mechanically swabbing the vagina, by using a syringe for lavage, or by the use of suppositories. In all studies of vaginal cleansing, babies are breastfed. In Malawi, the cleansing was done with chlorhexidine swabbing (Biggar 1996). In Kenya, vaginal cleansing is accomplished by using a syringe for lavage (Gaillard 1997).

A preliminary report from the Kenya group revealed that there was no significant difference in rates of transmission between the group using the lavage before breastfeeding and the control group; the research is ongoing. In the Côte d'Ivoire/Burkina Faso study, benzalkonium chloride vaginal suppositories are used daily at the end of pregnancy and at the onset of labor (Fowler 1997).

The trial completed in Malawi found little difference in transmission rates between groups that did or did not have vaginal swabbing. Biggar and colleagues (1996) reported that women had the birth canal, external genital area and infant's head cleansed every four hours once labor began. Babies whose mothers were treated were infected at a rate of 27 percent, very close to the 28 percent transmission rate of similar babies whose mothers received no treatment. There was, however, a significant difference with mothers whose membranes had ruptured more than four hours before delivery. In that case, only 25 percent of babies of treated mothers became HIV-infected, compared to 39 percent of babies of untreated mothers. Biggar also found that children whose mothers had vaginal cleansing had fewer infections of other types. Neonatal sepsis occurred in only 4.7 percent of the babies whose mothers had the vaginal cleansing, compared to 9.2 percent of the babies whose mothers did not.

Biggar provided various possible explanations for the relative ineffectiveness of vaginal cleansing in reducing HIV transmission, including the idea that babies were being infected via breastfeeding. He noted that infants infected soon after birth through HIV-contaminated colostrum or milk cannot be distinguished from infants infected in the birth canal.

## Risk Reduction Greater Than ACTG 076

Like Sullivan and Bell, who suggested the possibility of treating a population of untested women (with nevirapine or vitamin A), researchers in India examined interventions that might also be used with an untested population. Like Biggar, the Indian researchers used vaginal cleansing.

Ravinathan and colleagues (1996) combined three interventions. One intervention was to avoid "milking" the umbilical cord. Traditionally, people "milk" or squeeze the umbilical cord to force the blood into the baby before the cord is cut, so as to minimize anemia. The second intervention involved vaginal washing with a betadine one-percent solution during labor. The third intervention was avoidance of breastfeeding. The researchers employed vaginal washing and prevented umbilical cord milking for all mothers but restricted breastfeeding only for the HIV-positive women.

Their results were an impressive reduction in the rate of mother-to-child transmission from 38 percent among comparable untreated women to only 6 percent among treated women. The famous ACTG 076 reduced transmission by 67 percent, from 25 percent to 8 percent. Ravinathan's protocol reduced transmission by 84 percent, from 38 percent to 6 percent for comparable women. And it achieved the 84 percent reduction without antiretroviral drugs or cesareans. This study group was different from Biggar's in that vaginal cleansing was followed with restriction of breastfeeding. Ravinathan concluded:

> This type of perinatal care of vaginal washings, excluding milking of the umbilical cord during labor and restricting breastfeeding may be a promising approach since it could be recommended for all women irrespective of the HIV status and would not require an HIV counseling and testing infrastructure.

The wider ramifications of such a statement are enormous. These Indian researchers are suggesting the possibility of restricting the breastfeeding of an entire population of untested women.

## Study of Breastfeeding Children

In a trial begun in 1992, researchers in Nairobi, Kenya, randomly assigned 409 HIV-positive mothers to breast or formula-feed their children (John 1997). Mothers are given counseling and time to consider whether they want to participate in a random assignment of infant feeding. The Nairobi researchers (Kreiss 1997) hope to answer three important questions: How frequently is HIV transmitted to breast versus formula-fed children? What are the rates of death and illness in breast and formula-fed children? What other factors correlate to HIV infection? Formula is supplied at no cost to mother-baby pairs who are randomly assigned to formula-feed. Mothers are encouraged to cup-feed the formula but also use bottles when away from home (John 1997).

In other studies HIV-positive mothers will receive AZT and then breast-feed. Van de Perre (1998) suggested that breastfeeding could erase the gain of antiretroviral treatment. The effect of AZT on breastfeeding women may be negligible, it may be beneficial or it may be detrimental. There may be a viral load rebound in breastmilk. If so, antiretroviral treatment would not be applicable to breastfeeding women.

A viral load rebound generally happens only after more prolonged treatment, but can happen with a shorter course of drugs. Shaffer (1998) reported that women who received the short-course AZT treatment in Thailand did not show rebounding viral loads at one month postpartum. Women will be tested at six months postpartum to see if their viral loads have rebounded at that time. Wiktor and colleagues from the collaborative project in Côte d'Ivoire reported in 1996 that, at that time, four women had completed a shortened regimen of AZT, with a median duration of 28 days (Wiktor 1996). The women's viral loads were reduced significantly during treatment, although statistically significant viral load rebound was seen after delivery. In one of the four women, the viral load was more than twice her level at enrollment in the study. Thus she was breastfeeding during the time her viral load was rebounding, and this may have increased the relative risk of her transmitting the virus in her milk.

Until the trials are completed, it is conjecture to suggest how women's HIV viral loads will react to various lengths of drug treatment. Researchers in Côte d'Ivoire will follow the women and children for two years. Women who follow the traditional pattern may continue breastfeeding well into the baby's second year of life, so transmission could still occur long after the AZT treatment has ended. In 1997, Wiktor suggested that the likelihood of transmission could be reduced if mothers taking AZT stop breastfeeding after the first three months (Wiktor 1997).

## But If Women Aren't Tested?

While there is a great deal of interest in the research trials with AZT and other interventions, the fact remains that very few pregnant women world-wide are tested for HIV. What will be the point of studying interventions if HIV-infected women are not identified? How can one apply public health calculations about breast or formula feeding to untested women? Without testing and counseling programs, only universal recommendations can be made. Universal vitamin supplements, universal nevirapine and universal labor and delivery recommendations might be considered safe enough (although someone has to pay for even the cheapest options), but without testing and counseling programs, infant feeding decisions in endemic areas pose a terrible dilemma.

In 1997 UNAIDS estimated that only 10 percent of all HIV-infected individuals in the world know that they are infected. In the resource-poor world, there has been almost no voluntary testing and counseling facilities; little outside funding has as yet appeared. Testing has been conducted only in research studies and for purposes of surveillance, involving very small population samples and often done without identifying any of the individuals tested.

Even where testing and counseling programs are available, they are often shunned. Numerous excerpts from the book *Kampala Women Getting By: Wellbeing in the Time of AIDS* (Wallman 1996) describe a very strong preference among Ugandan women not to know their HIV status. Pregnant women could go to Mulago or to the AIDS Information Centre for HIV diagnosis, but many do not go, because they fear they may have AIDS. People avoid diagnosis because they know AIDS has no cure. "A pervasive fear in obtaining treatment and/or diagnosis is that the sufferer will be told that he/she has AIDS, and this is information no one wants to receive" (Wallman 1996:185). Sexually transmitted diseases used to be known as "diseases of the brave" among men, but are now often presumed to be symptoms of AIDS. An herbalist relates that she treats pregnant women with AIDS but does not tell them that they have AIDS (Wallman:138). A spiritual healer treats babies with AIDS but does not tell the mothers that their babies have AIDS because she does not want to worry them (Wallman:137).

Many people who suspect that they are infected do not want to know. In some studies, groups of pregnant women who were HIV-infected were *less* likely to agree to testing than groups of uninfected women. This was true in Nairobi (Kiarie 1996) and in New York (Bateman 1995). Verkuyl (1995) described his feelings practicing obstetrics in Zimbabwe, with needle sticks and small punctures in re-sterilized gloves. He said that detecting a fungal infection between his toes or an ulcer in his mouth brought on a cold sweat and an empathy with patients who do not want to be tested. At a rural hospital in South Africa, only 2 percent of people who were HIV-positive knew their HIV status. Among 63 HIV-positive women in urban Kenya, only one knew she was infected (UNAIDS 1997). In Zimbabwe a "substantial number" of women prefer not to be tested for HIV (Henderson 1997).

In theory, women should know their HIV status and their partner's so they can avoid becoming infected and avoid infecting others, including future sexual partners and children. But with no treatments available and difficulties with male compliance with "safe sex," there hasn't seemed to be much point in being tested. It is understandable that women would not want to know if they were HIV-positive if they feared that they would be stigmatized, beaten or thrown out of their home.

A woman's resistance to testing may end when her child becomes symptomatic. The child's symptoms "tell" the woman that she is probably HIV-infected — that she has infected her child. The test, then, only confirms the worst.

The reluctance to accept testing seems to improve with increased familiarity. One of the oldest identified epidemics has been around Kigali, Rwanda. In 1986, 30 percent of women were HIV-infected at the time of childbirth (Bizmungu 1989). In 1988, almost 75 percent of the women said that they did not expect a supportive reaction after revealing the test result to their male partners. By 1991, the situation had improved. The most common reactions of the male partners were acceptance, understanding and sympathy. Still, 21 percent of the women did not tell their male partners the results of their HIV test (Keogh 1994).

A testing and counseling program at the Chris-Hani Baragwanath Hospital in South Africa has had very good results using a male nurse who counsels couples together. The counseling of couples has been much more effective than the previous strategy of counseling women alone. In the past, some counselors had encouraged women not to disclose their HIV status (Gray, personal communication). Counseling couples together is better because men and women talk about their HIV status and can talk about protecting their unborn child. Researchers who worked in a testing and counseling program in Rwanda also recommended that HIV counseling in high-prevalence areas should include both members of a couple (Allen 1992).

In India, when HIV/AIDS was new, the level of AIDS education and acceptance of testing was low. A study was conducted among 200 pregnant women in Pune, India (Kapila 1997). Fewer than half (48.5 percent) had any awareness of HIV. Of this half, only 67 percent knew that HIV can be transmitted sexually, and only 8.2 percent knew that mothers could transmit HIV to the babies. Among the 25 unmarried pregnant teens, only three had any awareness of HIV. Only one knew that HIV could be transmitted sexually. It has been noted that in India it is not customary for people to talk about sex.

The most optimistic part of the report from Pune is that 90 percent of the women agreed to HIV testing after being counseled, probably motivated by a concern for the baby. This incentive is likely to work better where health workers have something to offer pregnant HIV-infected woman. Some researchers have reported that women agreed to participate in clinical trials because they wanted free medical treatment for themselves and their children (Coutsoudis 1995). Because children are universally cherished, a desire to protect them may be the strongest inducement in the campaign to reduce HIV transmission (Bassett and Mhloyi 1994). But exploiting a woman's maternal instincts to accept testing will do more harm than good to her and her baby if she tests positive and her male partner rejects or abuses her.

## Insights from Experiences

Results from a pilot study in Côte d'Ivoire and Burkina Faso were somewhat heartening. With free testing and encouragement from social workers, 90 percent of pregnant women accepted the idea of the test, and 73 percent returned for the test results, 53 percent spontaneously and an additional 20 percent after a home visit. The researchers fear, however, that without free testing and the availability of social workers, testing and counseling programs would be less effective (Cartoux 1996).

A survey of five sites in Africa examined the acceptance rate, return rate to learn test results and acceptability of interventions (antiretroviral therapy or vitamin A). Acceptance rates of testing were generally high, but return rates were lower. Still, the overall acceptability rates were at least 70 percent. The most common reason given for refusing HIV testing was the need to consult with the partner. The recommendations included offering HIV services to adults and children, fighting against HIV discrimination and training health care professionals.

Rubini and colleagues (1998) noted that 42.9 percent of HIV-infected women were not identified. These women had children attending a Pediatric Immunology Clinic in Rio de Janeiro between 1995 and 1997. The fact that health care providers were not recommending testing or treatment reinforced the need to educate and train health providers.

Health providers who are aware of the benefits of testing and treating HIV-positive women have been able to help women by repeatedly exposing them to the idea of HIV testing. Matavou Somali of TASO, the AIDS Support Organization Uganda, reported good results with 20 women who had children attending a pediatric clinic in Kampala. Each time the women brought their children to the clinic, they were exposed to HIV counseling. At the end of three months, all women had consented to HIV testing, and nine of the 20 were HIV-infected. Of the nine, six agreed to use condoms to protect others. Among the eleven HIV-negative women, three opted to abstain from sex, and eight opted to use condoms until their partners agreed to take an HIV test (Somali 1997).

Many groups, including UNAIDS, strongly recommend that HIV testing be confidential, voluntary, and carried out within a counseling program. People have the right to decide whether they want to be tested and whether they want to obtain the results of their test. The purpose of testing should be to allow people to make their own decisions — even when pregnant. With mandatory screening pregnant women may simply avoid all prenatal care because they do not want to be tested. This is true for women in both industrialized and resource-poor countries. When women hear that they will be tested, some avoid health care workers, use the services of a traditional birth attendant or choose to receive no prenatal care. With excellent HIV counseling programs, almost all pregnant women consent to testing and mandatory measures are not needed.

In some countries, however, women are routinely tested for HIV without informed consent. Batterink (1994:49) reported this to be the case in Thailand. In the United States testing is supposed to be voluntary, although the state of New York has begun to test all newborn babies without consent. Since a test of the baby is a test of the mother, this is the first example in the United States of mandatory testing. Another major problem with the New York plan is that results are often not available for weeks. Some HIV-positive women are suing New York State because they would not have breastfed for weeks if they had been informed sooner that they were HIV-positive (McGovern 1998).

In resource-poor countries, rapid testing is useful, if problematic. It eliminates the problem of women failing to return weeks later to learn of the results, but rapid testing can steamroll women into taking a test before they have really had a chance to think about it. While rapid testing is quite cost-effective and accurate, and enables physicians to treat HIV-positive women, it may eliminate the truly voluntary nature of testing.

All testing programs, rapid or not, cost money. It remains to be seen how much funding governments or private foundations will make available to pay for testing and treatment programs in resource-poor countries. To date, few Westerners have focused much attention on mother-to-child HIV transmission in these countries. Likewise, few have paid much attention to how women around the world actually feed their babies.

---

# References

Allen, S., et al. 1992. Confidential HIV testing and condom promotion in Africa. *Journal of the American Medical Association* 268: 3338–3343.

Ammann, Arthur J. 1997. Setting worldwide goals for reducing transmission from mothers to infants. Presented at the Conference on Global Strategies for the Prevention of HIV Transmission from Mothers to Infants, Washington, D.C., September 3–6.

Bassett, M. T., and M. Mhloyi. 1994. Women and AIDS in Zimbabwe: The making of an epidemic. In *AIDS: The Politics of Survival*, eds. N. Krieger and G. Margo. Amityville, New York: Baywood, pp. 125–139.

Bateman, D. A. 1995. Newborn human immunodeficiency virus testing in New York: A legislative quandary. *Archives of Pediatric and Adolescent Medicine* 149: 582–583.

Batterink, Cisa, et al. 1994. *AIDS and Pregnancy: Reactions to Problems of HIV-positive Pregnant Women and their Children in Chiang Mai, Thailand.* Amsterdam: VU University Press.

Becquart, P., et al. 1998. Early postnatal mother-to-child transmission of HIV-1 in Bangui, Central African Republic. Presented at the Fifth Conference on Retroviruses and Opportunistic Infections, Chicago, Illinois, February 1–5.

Bell, Jensa, and Henry S. Sacks. 1997. Cost-effectiveness of vitamin A supplementation to reduce perinatal transmission of HIV in resource-poor countries. Presented at the Fourth Conference on Retroviruses and Opportunistic Infections, Washington, D.C., January 22–27. Abstract 291.

Biggar, Robert J., et al. 1996. Perinatal intervention trial in Africa: Effect of a birth canal cleansing intervention to prevent HIV transmission. *Lancet* 347: 1647–1650.

Bizmungu, C., et al. 1989. Nationwide community-based serological survey of HIV-1 and other human retrovirus infections. *Lancet* 335: 941-943.

Blanche, S., et al. 1989. A prospective study of perinatal infection of infants born to women seropositive for human immunodeficiency virus type 1. *New England Journal of Medicine* 320: 1643–1648.

Bulterys, M., A. Chao, A. Dushimimana and A. Saah. 1996. Fatal complications after cesarean section in HIV-infected women. *AIDS* 10: 923–924.

Burger, Harold, et al. 1997. Maternal serum vitamin A levels are not associated with mother-to-child transmission of HIV-1 in the United States. *Journal of Acquired Immune Deficiency Syndromes* 14: 321–326.

Cartoux, Michel, et al. 1996. Acceptability of interventions to reduce mother-to-child transmission of HIV-1 in West Africa. *Journal of Acquired Immune Deficiency Syndromes* 12: 290–292.

_____, et al. 1998. Acceptability of voluntary HIV counseling and testing (VCT) and interventions to reduce mother-to-child transmission of HIV in Africa. Twelfth World AIDS Conference, Geneva, Switzerland, June 28–July 3. Abstract 23310.

Chun, Tae-Wook, et al. 1997. Presence of an inducible HIV-1 latent reservoir during highly active antiretroviral therapy. *Proceedings of the National Academy of Sciences* 94: 13193–13197.

Connor, E. M., et al. 1994. Reduction of maternal-infant transmission of human immunodeficiency virus type 1 with zidovudine therapy. *New England Journal of Medicine* 331: 1173–1180.

Coutsoudis, Anna, et al. 1995. The effects of vitamin A supplementation on the morbidity of children born to HIV-infected women. *American Journal of Public Health* 85: 1076–1081.

European Collaborative Study. 1994. Cesarean section and risk of vertical transmission of HIV-1 infection. *Lancet* 343: 1464–1467.

———. 1996. Vertical transmission of HIV-1: Maternal immune status and obstetric factors. *AIDS* 10: 1675–1681.

Fawzi, Wafaie. 1998. A randomized trial of vitamin supplements in relation to pregnancy outcomes and T-cell counts among HIV-infected women in Tanzania. Presented at the Twelfth World AIDS Conference, Geneva, Switzerland, June 28–July 3. Abstract 42475.

Feinman, Jane. 1997. Tackling mother-to-child HIV in Côte d'Ivoire. *Lancet* 350: 1084.

Fowler, Mary Glenn. 1997. Update on International Trials to Prevent HIV Transmission from Mothers to Infants. Presented at the Conference on Global Strategies for the Prevention of HIV Transmission from Mothers to Infants, Washington, D.C., September 3–6.

Gabiano, Clara, et al. 1992. Mother-to-child transmission of HIV type 1: Risk of infection and correlates of transmission. *Pediatrics* 90: 69–74.

Gaillard, Philippe, et al. 1997. Cervico-vaginal lavage with chlorhexidine during childbirth to reduce mother-to-child transmission of HIV-1, Mombasa, Kenya. Presented at the Conference on Global Strategies for the Prevention of HIV Transmission from Mothers to Infants, Washington, D.C., September 3–6.

Gomez, M. Perry, et al. 1997. Zidovudine reduces vertical transmission of HIV in the Bahamas. Presented at the Conference on Global Strategies for the Prevention of HIV Transmission from Mothers to Infants, Washington, D.C., September 3–6.

Gray, Glenda E. 1998. Personal communication to author.

Henderson, Charles W. 1997. Breastfeeding still supported despite AIDS pandemic. *AIDS Weekly Plus*, August 18, p. 24.

Ho, David. 1998. Residual pool of HIV after prolonged combination therapy. Presented at the Fifth Conference on Retroviruses and Opportunistic Infections, Chicago, Illinois, February 1–5.

John, Grace. 1997. Epidemiology of HIV-1 transmission through breastfeeding. Presented at the Conference on Affordable Options for the Prevention of Mother-to-Child Transmission of HIV-1, Johannesburg, South Africa, November 19–20.

Joint Statement by CDC, UNAIDS, NIH and ANRS. 1998. (Following the) Announcement by the Ministry of Public Health of Thailand and the CDC of Results from Their Mother-to-Child Transmission Trial, February 20.

Kapila, Bharucha, M. Ambekar and K. Khatri. 1997. Pretest counseling and HIV testing at antenatal clinic — Pune, India. Presented at the Conference on Global Strategies for the Prevention of HIV Transmission from Mothers to Infants, Washington, D.C., September 3–6.

Keogh, P., et al. 1994. The social impact of HIV infection on women in Kigali, Rwanda: A prospective study. *Social Science and Medicine* 38 (8): 1047–1053.

Kiarie, J., et al. 1996. Acceptability of antenatal HIV-1 screening. Presented at the Eleventh International Conference on AIDS, Vancouver, Canada, July 7–9. Abstract Mo.C.211.

Kind, Christine, et al. 1998. Prevention of vertical HIV transmission: Additive protective effect of elective Cesarean section and zidovudine prophylaxis. *AIDS* 12: 205–210.

Kreiss, J. 1997. Breastfeeding and vertical transmission of HIV-1. *Acta Paediatrica Supplement* 421: 113–117.

Krivine, A., S. Le Bourdelles, G. Firtion and P. Lebon. 1997. Viral kinetics in HIV-1 perinatal infection. *Lancet* 350: 493.

Kuhn, Louise, et al. 1996. Cesarean deliveries and maternal-infant HIV transmission: Results from a prospective study in South Africa. *Journal of Acquired Immune Deficiency Syndrome Retrovirology* 11: 478–483.

_____. 1997. Timing of maternal-infant HIV transmission: Associations between intrapartum factors and early polymerase chain reaction results. *AIDS* 11: 429–435.

Landesman, Sheldon H., et al. 1996. Obstetrical factors and the transmission of human immunodeficiency virus type 1 from mother to child. *New England Journal of Medicine* 334: 1617–1623.

Maguire, A., et al. 1997. Potential risk factors for vertical HIV-1 transmission in Catalonia, Spain: The protective role of Cesarean section. *AIDS* 11: 1851–1857.

Mandelbrot, Laurent, et al. 1998. Perinatal HIV-1 transmission. *Journal of the American Medical Association* 280: 55–60.

McDonald, A., et al. 1996. Perinatal exposure to HIV in Australia, 1982–1995. Presented at the Annual Conference by Australia's Society for HIV Medicine, Sydney, Australia, November 14–17.

McGovern, Theresa M. 1998. Lawsuit demands return of "baby AIDS" test results to mothers within 48 hours. New York: HIV Law Project, May 14.

Nduati, Ruth W., Grace C. John and Barbara A. Richardson. 1995. Human immunodeficiency virus type 1-infected cells in breast milk: Association with immunosupression and vitamin A deficiency. *Journal of Infectious Diseases* 172: 1461–1468.

Nicoll, Angus, and Marie-Louise Newell. 1996. Preventing perinatal transmission of HIV: The effect of breast-feeding (letter). *Journal of the American Medical Association* 276: 1552

Office of Public Health and Science, HHS. 1997. *U.S. Public Health Service Recommendations for Use of Antiretroviral Drugs During Pregnancy for Maternal Health and Reduction of Perinatal Transmission of Human Immunodeficiency Virus Type 1 in the United States.* Washington, D.C.: U.S. Government Printing Office.

Peckham, C., and M.-L. Newell. 1997. Human immunodeficiency virus infection and mode of delivery. *Acta Paediatrica Supplement* 421: 104–106.

Piot, Peter. 1997. The global status and response to the epidemic. Presented at the Fourth Conference on Retroviruses and Opportunistic Infections, Washington, D.C., January 22–27.

Pizzo, Philip A., and Catherine M. Wilfert. 1995. Perspectives on pediatric human immunodeficiency virus infections. *Pediatric Infectious Disease Journal* 14: 536.

Ravinathan, Ramanathan, et al. 1996. Prevention of mother-to-child transmission through perinatal care. Presented at the Eleventh International Conference on AIDS, Vancouver, Canada, July 7–12. Abstract We.C.3580.

Rubini, Norma P. M., et al. 1998. Main difficulties in the reduction of HIV vertical transmission in Rio de Janeiro, Brazil. Presented at the Twelfth World AIDS Conference, Geneva, Switzerland, June 28–July 3. Abstract 23311.

Semba, Richard D., et al. 1994. Maternal vitamin A deficiency and mother-to-child transmission of HIV-1. *Lancet* 343:1593–1597.

_____. 1998. Vitamin A supplementation and human immunodeficiency virus load in injection drug users. *Journal of Infectious Diseases* 177: 611–616.

Shaffer, Nathan. 1998. Randomized placebo-controlled trial of short-course oral ZDV to reduce perinatal HIV transmission. Presented at the Twelfth World AIDS Conference, Geneva, Switzerland, June 28–July 3. Abstract 33163.

Somali, Matavou. 1997. HIV counseling as a guiding factor to prevention of HIV infection from mother to child. Presented at the Conference on Global Strategies for the Prevention of HIV Transmission from Mothers to Infants, Washington, D.C., September 3–6.

Staple, D. G., N. Khithani and J. K. Maniar. 1997. Role of AZT Prophylaxis in Vertical Transmission of HIV. Presented at the Conference on Global Strategies for the Prevention of HIV Transmission from Mothers to Infants, Washington, D.C., September 3–6.

Stoltzfus, Rebecca J., et al. 1993. High dose vitamin A supplementation of breastfeeding Indonesian mothers: Effects on the vitamin A status of mother and infant. *Journal of Nutrition* 123: 666–675.

Sullivan, John. 1997. Perinatal transmission and early virus replication events in babies. Presented at the Fourth International Conference on Retroviruses and Opportunistic Infections, Washington, D.C., January 22–27.

UNAIDS Joint United Nations Programme on HIV/AIDS. 1996. UNAIDS announces new clinical trials for the prevention of mother-to-child transmission of HIV. Press release, Geneva, Switzerland: UNAIDS, July 9.

_____. 1997. *Report on the Global HIV/AIDS Epidemic.* Geneva, Switzerland: UNAIDS.

_____. 1998. International meeting calls for concerted action to prevent mother-to-child transmission of HIV. Press release, Geneva, Switzerland, March 24.

Van de Perre, Philippe, Deo-Gratis Hitimana, Philippe Lepage. 1988. Human immunodeficiency virus antibodies of IgG, IgA, and IgM subclasses in milk of seropositive mothers. *Journal of Pediatrics* 113 (6): 1039–1041.

Verkuyl, Douwe A. A. 1995. Practicing obstetrics and gynaecology in areas with a high prevalence of HIV infection. *Lancet* 346: 293–296.

Waldholz, Michael. 1998. AZT price cut for Third World mothers-to-be. *Wall Street Journal*, March 5, p. B1.

Wallman, Sandra. 1996. *Kampala Women Getting By: Wellbeing in the Time of AIDS.* London: James Currey Ltd.

Waloch, Marek, et al. 1997. Retrospective and prospective study of children born to HIV symptomatic mothers and consequences. Presented at the Conference on Global Strategies for the Prevention of HIV Transmission from Mothers to Infants, Washington, D.C., September 3–6.

Wiktor, Stefan Z., E. R. Ekpini and T. S. Sibailly. 1996. The effectiveness of oral zidovudine administration late pregnancy in lowering plasma and cervicov-aginal HIV-1 viral load in HIV-infected women in Abidjan, Côte d'Ivoire. Pre-sented at the Eleventh International Conference on AIDS, Vancouver, Canada, July 7–12. Abstract TU.C. 443.

Wiktor, Stefan Z. 1997. Trial in Côte d'Ivoire. Presented at the Tenth Conference on HIV and STDs in Africa, Abidjan, Côte d'Ivoire, December 7–11.

# PART TWO:

## *Breastfeeding Questions*

CHAPTER FOUR

―――――――

# Won't More Babies Die
# Without Breastfeeding?

A central question is how babies living under the worst conditions will do if they are not breastfed. On the one hand, it seems unthinkable to recommend that some Third World women might totally avoid breastfeeding. It brings to mind images of Third World babies being given dirty baby bottles containing overdiluted formula or foods totally unsuitable for babies. It brings to mind images of babies becoming so malnourished that they finally die of infections that should not have been fatal. Breastfeeding is much more than a feeding method; it is an integral part of the interaction between mothers and babies. In resource-poor countries, breastfeeding has been a health and economic necessity.

On the other hand, breastmilk from HIV-infected mothers clearly can transmit the virus. The challenge to public health officials will be to make infant feeding recommendations, considering the varying circumstances, for HIV-infected mothers. But ultimately mothers will make their own decisions, and, as this chapter will show, mothers often disregard advice about infant feeding.

Westerners may enter discussions about Third World infant feeding and HIV as gatekeepers; that is, they may help decide which, if any, alternatives to breastfeeding to support.

There are several erroneous notions that permeate First World discussions about Third World infant feeding. One is that most young babies in resource-poor countries are being fed only breastmilk, and that their baseline health is typical of what one reads about children exclusively breastfed. Another mistaken notion is that women either breast or bottle-feed, and that these are two distinct patterns. A third myth is that any amount of breast-feeding keeps babies healthy, no matter what else they are fed. This chapter covers breastfeeding research, which, though far from conclusive, might help educate uninformed Westerners.

## Breastfeeding Research?

Those from other disciplines may not be aware of the complexity of breastfeeding research. Breastfeeding, after all, sounds so straightforward. Women put their babies to breast and give them perfect food, complete with immunoglobulins and other protective factors. But the research is remarkably broad in scope, offering many insights beyond the common presentations on the benefits of exclusive breastfeeding.

The benefits of exclusive breastfeeding are, nevertheless, truly remark-able (American Academy of Pediatrics 1997, Akré 1989, Cunningham 1991, Lawrence 1994). Exclusively breastfed babies have the lowest rates of mortal-ity and morbidity, have many fewer gastrointestinal illnesses (Brown 1989) and suffer much less diarrheal disease (Scott-Emuakpor 1986). Moreover, exclusively breastfed babies have fewer episodes of bacteremia-meningitis (Takala 1989) and experience fewer respiratory illnesses (Lanner 1990) and ear infections (Duncan 1993, Teele 1989, Kero 1987). Exclusively breastfed babies have fewer episodes of wheezing (Merrett 1988) and other allergic symptoms (Savilahti 1987, Saarinen 1995) and are less likely to die from infant botulism (Arnon 1986) and SIDS (Cunningham 1995). Older children and adults who were exclusively breastfed as infants have lower rates of celiac disease (Greco 1988), Crohn's disease (Koletzko 1989), lymphoma (Davis 1988) and insulin dependent diabetes (Karjalainen 1992).

The World Health Organization (1996) recommends exclusive breast-feeding for the first four to six months, and suggests that, afterward, children continue to be breastfed while receiving appropriate complimentary foods for up to 2 years of age and beyond (WHO 1996). There is clear evidence that compliance with these two major recommendations results in mortality reduc-tion. It is because supplemented breastfeeding offers significantly less protec-tion that the World Health Organization (1996) and UNICEF (Barrington-Ward 1997) recommend so strongly that early breastfeeding be exclusive. Some papers from the WHO (World Health Assembly 1994) and from UNICEF (Bel-lamy 1998:28) recommend that women extend exclusive breastfeeding for a full six months if possible. The American Academy of Pediatrics (1997) rec-ommends six months of exclusive breastfeeding with continuing breastfeed-ing "for at least 12 months and thereafter for as long as mutually desirable."

## Types of Dialogue About Infant Feeding

That *research* dialogue is not the same as *advocacy* dialogue is a point that needs emphasizing. Dr. Penny Van Esterik, a professor of anthropology and breastfeeding advocate, has noted that advocacy discourse and research discourse offer very different frameworks for interpreting the controversy over infant formula (Van Esterik 1989:15). Even to researchers in other fields (such as HIV research), breastfeeding advocacy language is probably more familiar than breastfeeding research language.

Both forms of discourse have much to offer in discussions about HIV and infant feeding. But they are different, and advocacy dialogue should not crowd out research dialogue. Breastfeeding-advocacy dialogue has been important in pointing out the aggressive marketing schemes of the formula companies in resource-poor countries. In chapter six, the Nestlé boycott and the WHO Code of Marketing, clearly two important issues, are discussed.

It should be noted that advocacy for breastfeeding has not necessarily been the same as advocacy for Third World women. The gap grew even larger when HIV turned mothers' milk from the most benevolent substance imaginable into something potentially deadly. To advocate for universal breastfeeding is not the same as to advocate for women's right to make their own informed infant feeding decisions. Even before HIV, many felt that the breastfeeding-advocacy position was different from a woman's-advocacy position. Breastfeeding author Pam Carter (1995:234) opined that, in their efforts to "save" breastfeeding, First and Third World policymakers acted as if Third World women were objects to be saved from capitalism, rather than people who might know something about their own situations. Some impassioned First World statements imply that, left in the care of their mothers, half of all non-breastfed babies die, and that it is up to others to save these babies. If the women involved were surveyed and listened to, they would have the opportunity to explain other aspects of their lives.

## The Reality of Contemporary Infant Feeding

Many research reports document that even for the youngest babies, exclusive breastfeeding is not the common pattern. In addition, some mothers who say that they are breastfeeding exclusively, when asked again, often admit that they are giving other liquids or semisolids (Hanson 1986, Haider 1996b, Greiner 1997a). For example, Haider talked to Bangladeshi mothers whose babies were hospitalized with diarrheal disease. Some of these mothers said that they were feeding only breastmilk, but it is counterintuitive that exclusively breastfed babies would have such severe diarrhea as to require hospitalization. On further questioning, *all* mothers admitted that they were not breastfeeding exclusively. Hence the diarrhea and the hospitalization.

Mothers in Istanbul claimed that they were breastfeeding exclusively, but the researchers who observed them saw that they were not (Koctürk and Zetterström 1988). Anthropologists working in the field in 11 countries observed that mothers occasionally said that they gave their babies only breastmilk at the very same moment they were casually putting other foods into their babies' mouths. "Only mothers know that weaning is always and that mixed-feeding is the method" (Raphael and Davis 1985:143).

Many other researchers have reported that mixed-feeding — not exclusive breastfeeding — is the common pattern and has been for decades (Boerma 1991, David 1984, Dimond 1987, Grantham-McGregor 1970, Latham 1996, McLaren 1966). This is the case even in the most poorly resourced countries. While most women do breastfeed, most also feed their babies other liquids and semisolids.

In industrialized countries such as the United States, mixed-fed babies who get breastmilk and properly prepared infant formula do well, although not as well as exclusively breastfed babies (Scariati 1997). The more breastmilk the babies receive, the healthier they are.

In resource-poor counties, many young mixed-fed babies get one very good food (breastmilk) plus varying amounts of not-so-good supplements, and the quality of the latter makes a significant difference. A "breastfed" baby who is supplemented with small amounts of cereal would be expected to be much healthier than a "breastfed" baby who is supplemented with many contaminated bottles.

With toddlers and young babies, the quality of other items in the diet is particularly significant. A study of Bangladeshi children under 24 months of age showed that children who received no breastmilk at all were four times more likely to die than those who were still partially breastfeeding (Teka 1996). Mothers who were illiterate and very poor were more likely to be feeding their toddlers inadequate amounts of inappropriate foods, and mortality risk increased with severe malnutrition. This report is similar to Lepage's 1981 report from Rwanda that partially breastfed children (aged 0–23 months) had a survival rate three times higher than those who had completely stopped breastfeeding.

## Mixed-Feeding Throughout the World

Like mothers all over the world, mothers in Africa combine breast and bottle-feeding. The practice is not new. Archeologists have found ancient feeding vessels that date from the tenth century b.c.e. and from many centuries thereafter. Among ruins from the ninth century b.c.e. scientists found a depiction of a woman with a very modern-looking baby bottle (Brennemann 1923:622). Mothers in east Africa in 1912 withheld colostrum and supplemented breastfeeding from the beginning (McLaren 1966). From the end of the first month, they fed their babies thin soups and other foods that included cow and goat milk. East African shops offered feeding bottles for sale in 1912.

Today, even in resource-poor countries, breastfeeding is not so solid a practice as it may seem. Health workers in Uganda recommended that women be given breastfeeding education at each of their infrequent prenatal visits (Wellstart 1994). At a 1996 conference in Durban, South Africa, it was noted, "exclusive breastfeeding in Africa, or elsewhere is rare" (Humphrey 1996). Exclusive breastfeeding was described as almost nonexistent in Bangladesh (Haider 1996a). The situation in Senegal in 1992 was described as "a complete absence of exclusive breastfeeding" (Cantrelle 1971). Researchers in Kenya coined the term "early triple nipple feeding" to describe the common pattern of supplementing early breastfeeding with bottle-feeding (Latham 1986). Zerfas (1990) also noted that exclusive breastfeeding in Kenya was uncommon.

Outside of Africa, exclusive breastfeeding is also uncommon. Only 4 percent of mothers in Al-Ain, the United Arab Emirates, practiced exclusive breastfeeding in the first month (al-Mazroui 1997). In Puerto Rico, Panchula (1998) noted that "NO ONE even remembers seeing a child who was exclusively breastfed." Although mothers in Haiti believe that breastfeeding is best for babies, mixed-feeding is the norm. People there see bottle-feeding as an unavoidable adaptation to worsening economic conditions that make it necessary for women to travel long distances to earn a living (Coreil 1998). Younger mothers in Haiti see bottle-feeding as modern and convenient.

Titles of medical journal articles include the following: "Has the bottle battle been lost?" (Boerma 1991) and "The Rarity of the exclusively breastfed infant" (Dimond 1987). A research monograph from Wellstart is entitled "A Breastfeeding Culture Without Exclusive Breastfeeding in Lesotho" (Latham and Almroth 1996).

Although the Koran advises Moslem women to breastfeed for two years, many rural Moslem women have been observed to stop early or refuse entirely to breastfeed. Those who stopped early used explanations that could be justified, such as saying that their milk supply was "finished" (Azaiza 1995, Zurayk 1981).

The World Health Organization (1996) reported that exclusive breastfeeding rates were two percent in Nigeria, two percent in Ghana, three percent in urban Zambia and four percent in rural Zambia.

Representatives from Wellstart, UNICEF, and the United States Agency for International Development (USAID) participated in a 1992 feasibility evaluation of a protocol that might have studied mother-to-child transmission of HIV in Rwanda (Wellstart 1994). Their 1994 evaluation noted how difficult it would be to get mothers to breastfeed, or bottle-feed, exclusively, since most mothers breastfeed but also give supplements. It would be impossible to get accurate results about the rate of HIV transmission if "breastfeeding mothers" also bottle-fed, and especially if "bottle-feeding" mothers also offered the breast. The Wellstart report (1994:4) noted, "A principal issue was the difficulty of getting *exclusive* practice of either of these behaviors." Rwanda is listed as being the country with the world's highest percentage of exclusive breastfeeding, at 90 percent, but the people in the field from Wellstart, USAID and UNICEF did not find high rates of exclusive breastfeeding. In any case, researchers canceled the proposed study in Rwanda when war broke out in April 1994.

## Research from Intermediate Countries

Health officials within countries (and Western analysts) would find it useful to know what percentage of babies die, based on how the children are fed. But quantifying death rates among babies in resource-poor countries is close to impossible. There has never been a study to compare mortality rates among breastfed or bottle-fed babies in Africa, for example. Research now being conducted in Nairobi, Kenya, will be the first to describe the health of formula-fed babies in an urban area of a resource-poor country.

Meanwhile, there are reports from intermediate countries about non-HIV-related mortality. Clavanno's 1982 report from the Philippines was that 2.46 percent of the bottle-fed babies died, compared to 0.03 percent of the exclusively breastfed babies and 0.16 percent of babies who were fed by both breast and bottle. However, 77.6 percent of the babies who died were of low birthweight. Low birthweight babies often have a weak suck and are more likely to end up in the bottle-feeding group. The groups, then, were not comparable. While the 2.46 percent death rate among bottle-fed babies is significant, it is lower by a factor of ten to twenty than the death rates for babies who are breastfed by HIV-positive mothers.

In a report from Malaysia (Habicht 1986), the calculated risk associated with total lack of breastfeeding was to add 25 extra deaths per 1000 in the first six months. While this mortality risk is significant, it too is ten to twenty times lower than the mortality rate expected for babies who are breastfed by HIV-positive mothers.

Most infant feeding studies do not have comparable groups of mother-baby pairs in the breast and bottle-feeding groups. Mothers who self-select to breast or bottle-feed are often different in terms of demographics and the need to work outside the home. In almost all studies, there has been no attempt to control the number of low birth weight babies who end up in any particular feeding group. In reality, many small babies who do not suck strongly end up in the bottle-feeding group. These small babies tend to be sick more.

Breastfeeding research studies have also been plagued by problems with definitions, which have weakened the validity of some conclusions. In a few studies, partially breastfed babies are called "non-breastfed" and are included with the bottle-fed babies. Researchers Acheson and Truelove (1961) correlated the way that babies were fed with how likely they were to develop ulcerative colitis later in life. In their attention to babies' colons, these researchers were strict with definitions: "A patient was regarded as having ceased to be breast-fed as soon as artificial feeding was started. Thus a period during which breast-feeding was supplemented by artificial feeds did not count as breast-feeding."

When Ryder (1991) evaluated transmission rates among babies of HIV-positive mothers in Zaire, he also referred to the mixed-fed (breast and bottle) babies as "non-breastfed." He found that "non-breastfed" babies (including partially breastfed babies) had more non-HIV related illnesses than exclusively breastfed babies had. Young (1982), in Tunisia, also labeled breastfed babies who received supplements as "non-breastfed."

But in most studies, babies are classified as "breastfed" if they receive *any* breastmilk (Heinig and Dewey 1996). A baby who is breastfed even once is placed in the same category as a baby who is breastfed exclusively for six months.

The practice of including these "ever breastfed" babies with exclusively breastfed babies tends to dramatically underrepresent the benefits of exclusive breastfeeding. Some researchers have even concluded, incorrectly, that breastfeeding does not save lives. Dugdale (1971) reported research from Kuala Lumpur, Malaysia: "Breast-feeding appears to offer no advantages over artificial feeding." But his "breastfed" babies were mixed-fed. Glass and colleagues (1986) concluded that breastfeeding offered little or no protection against rotavirus diarrhea in Bangladesh. But they defined breastfeeding "to include those children receiving breast-milk along with food supplements." So their unfavorable reports about "breastfeeding" are not valid criticisms. By contrast, Clemens and colleagues (1993) did differentiate between partial and exclusive breastfeeding in Bangladesh. They found that exclusive breastfeeding was associated with significant protection against severe rotavirus.

## Definitions of Breastfeeding

Although it is commonly recommended that researchers distinguish between different types of breastfeeding, many failed to do so. Even now, some consider it nit-picking to distinguish between "exclusive breastfeeding without water" and "almost exclusive breastfeeding with water." After all, one might argue, with other diets the addition of water is irrelevant. But, as the World Health Organization (1996) has noted, the water is often unclean, and the addition of plain water increases the chances of a baby suffering from diarrhea. When breastfed babies in the Philippines were given supplemental water, this doubled and tripled the likelihood of diarrhea (Popkin 1990).

Years ago, when some researchers reported that breastfeeding provided great protection and other researchers reported that breastfeeding provided no protection at all, the need for clear definitions became obvious. So members of the Interagency Group for Action on Breastfeeding met in 1988 to standardize definitions of breastfeeding (Labbok and Krasovec 1990). This group noted that full breastfeeding can be "exclusive breastfeeding," by which babies receive nothing but breastmilk, not even vitamins or water, or "almost exclusive breastfeeding," which allows for the infrequent consumption of water, vitamins, minerals or juice. "Partial breastfeeding" can be high, medium or low, depending on the frequency or percentage of other liquids or solids fed to babies. "High partial breastfeeding" refers to babies who receive more than 80 percent of their feeds from breastmilk. This is a very common pattern in resource-poor countries. "Token breastfeeding" refers to babies who consume breastmilk irregularly or for comfort and not for nutrition.

In 1991 the World Health Organization also convened a meeting to assess breastfeeding practices and came up with its own set of definitions. "Exclusive breastfeeding" allows a breastfed baby to receive vitamins, mineral supplements or medicines. "Predominant breastfeeding" refers to breastfed babies who also receive water, or water-based drinks such as teas, fruit juices and vitamins, minerals or medicines. "Complementary feeding" refers to children who consume breastmilk plus other semisolid foods or other nonhuman milks.

Labbok and colleagues (1997) prefer their definitions from the Interagency Group for Action on Breastfeeding, pointing out that the Interagency Group's definitions are based on biological impact, on both baby and mother. This is particularly important in discussing the fertility reducing benefits associated with breastfeeding. Women in the first six months postpartum are unlikely to become pregnant under "exclusive breastfeeding," "almost exclusive breastfeeding" and "high partial breastfeeding." On the other hand, the World Health Organization definition of "predominant breastfeeding" allows unlimited amounts of water and juices. These cannot only expose babies to contaminants, they also can reduce the amount of sucking time.

If babies suck on bottles, even to take water, they are often less interested in sucking on their mothers' nipples. If babies suck less on their mothers' nipples, their mothers are more likely to resume menstruating and ovulating. It is nipple stimulation that keeps women infertile.

## Great Benefits with Exclusive Breastfeeding

Although there have been many more studies about morbidity differences between breast and bottle-fed babies, comparisons of mortality are more relevant to discussions about AIDS. Dr. Cesar Victora's (1987) oft-quoted report of babies in urban Brazil showed that exclusive breastfeeding offered great protection against mortality. Total lack of breastfeeding increased the risk of diarrheal death fourteenfold, compared to babies who were exclusively breastfed. Total lack of breastfeeding increased the risk of death from respiratory infections three and one-half fold, compared to babies who were exclusively breastfed. With other causes of death (meningitis, skin infections, measles, whooping cough, tuberculosis), mortality for nonbreastfed babies was two and one-half times greater.

Feachem and Koblinsky (1984) limited their analysis to consideration of diarrhea only. They analyzed other researchers' studies of diarrheal disease and noted that, in terms of mortality, there were nine studies from five countries (England, the United States, Canada, Sweden and Egypt) to review. From these studies conducted between 1884 and 1980, they concluded that babies who received no breastmilk were 25 times more likely to die from diarrhea than exclusively breastfed babies were.

The differences in mortality rates reported by Victora and by Feachem and Koblinsky are dramatic for two reasons. First, these particular figures refer to the two (uncommon) extremes of exclusive breastfeeding and exclusive bottle-feeding. Secondly, these dramatic statistics involve diarrhea. Diarrhea studies present breastfeeding at its best. But diarrhea is not even the most common cause of death in children under five; it is second to pneumonia (Division of Child Health 1998). But since breastfeeding looks less protective in pneumonia studies, diarrhea studies are the ones most frequently referred to.

In 1997, in two different analyses of HIV and infant feeding, the researchers (Kahn 1997, Kuhn and Stein 1997) chose not to use either of the above mentioned diarrhea-focused analyses. Rather, they selected work that looked at death from all causes. They chose work done by Habicht and colleagues (1986) in Malaysia, who reported information on the mortality rates among more than five thousand children in Malaysia from 1940 to 1975. They found that babies who were exclusively breastfed (for an average duration of 1.7 months) enjoyed great protection. The researchers calculated that, if there had been no breastfeeding, twice as many babies would have died between 1 week and 1 year of age. The differences in mortality rates were much greater for children whose families lived under the worst conditions, lacking clean water and a flush toilet.

Yoon and colleagues (1996) followed 9942 children in the Philippines up to age 2 years. They found that 425 (4.3 percent) of all babies died. Bottle-fed babies, under the age of 6 months, were 8–10 times more likely to die from diarrhea, compared to breastfed babies. When diarrhea and respiratory infections were combined, bottle-fed babies were five times more likely to die in the first six months. For respiratory infections alone, however, the risk of death did not increase. The differences were greatest for low-birthweight babies and for babies whose mothers had the least formal education. The protective effects of breastfeeding were significant in the first six months of babies' lives.

Plank and Milanesi (1973) studied infant mortality among 1712 mother-baby pairs in rural Chile. They found that there were three times as many deaths among babies given bottles before the age of 3 months, compared to babies who were exclusively breastfed.

## Mixed-Feeding Scores Closer to No-Breastfeeding

The need to study mixed-feeding was not always apparent. But as AIDS is causing some women to abandon their traditional feeding patterns, this change compels us to ask how much of a mortality difference is likely with a switch from mixed-feeding to exclusive bottle-feeding. Suddenly, mixed-feeding warrants more attention.

Studies about infant feeding in intermediate countries typically find that mixed-feeding offers a level of protection much lower than exclusive breastfeeding, but not quite so bad as a total lack of breastfeeding. Mixed-feeding in intermediate countries typically scores closer to nonbreastfeeding than to exclusive breastfeeding. But since different studies find varying results, mixed-feeding scores better in some studies than in others.

Victora (1987) in urban Brazil found that, although mixed-feeding did not offer nearly as much protection against mortality as exclusive breastfeeding, it offered fairly good protection. The mortality rate for diarrhea was 4.2 times greater among those who received no breastmilk than among those who were mixed-fed. The mortality rate for respiratory infection was 1.6 times greater for those who received no breastmilk. But the mortality rate with other infections (measles, meningitis, tuberculosis, whooping cough) was actually higher for those who were mixed-fed. With these illnesses, mixed-fed babies had more than twice the risk of dying compared to children who received no breastmilk.

Habicht, Da Vanzo and Butz (1986) found mixed-feeding in Malaysia to be less protective than what Victora had reported from Brazil. Habicht and colleagues observed that, under the worst of home conditions (no piped water and no flush toilet), each month of mixed-feeding reduced only 0.8 infant deaths per 1000 live births, compared to a reduction of 5.5 deaths per 1000 live births with exclusive breastfeeding.

In their meta-analysis about the effects of diarrhea, Feachem and Koblinsky also found that mixed-feeding offered a much lower level of protection. For mortality, they had considered all the studies available (from Canada, England, Sweden, and the United States, 1884–1947, and Egypt, 1979–1980). Feachem and Koblinsky stated that all these studies contain severe methodological flaws and should be regarded as merely indicative. Even though they restricted their analysis to diarrhea (which should present breastfeeding at its best), they found that the protective value of mixed-feeding was less than one-eighth the protection offered by exclusive breastfeeding.

Plank and Milanesi (1973) pointed out that only when researchers observe the subjects can they assess the value of various feeding methods. Researchers need to know how many infant deaths took place during periods of exclusive breastfeeding, how many deaths during mixed-feeding and how many during exclusive bottle-feeding.

The benefit of knowing how many deaths happen under different feeding regimes may seem obvious, but researchers have not collected such information. Hobcraft's 1985 analysis, for example, is frequently cited as proving the benefits of breastfeeding. What Hobcraft actually studied was birth intervals — how long women went between subsequent births. He then estimated how long women had probably breastfed. So while Hobcraft's study showed that children are healthier if they are not born too soon after a sibling, it provided absolutely no information about the health of children during periods of exclusive breastfeeding, mixed-feeding or no breastfeeding.

Plank and Milanesi, observing the deaths as they occurred, found that mixed-feeding was not at all protective in their population of 1712 babies in rural Chile. Mixed-feeding was actually associated with a slightly higher rate of infant mortality (86.5 deaths per 1000 persons) than exclusive bottle-feeding (84.5 deaths per 1000 persons). There was no evidence that the continuation of breastfeeding offered any protection after the infants were given milk-based supplements. The authors suggested that exclusive breastfeeding was protective because it avoided the problems associated with bottle-feeding.

This finding has some similarity to an old morbidity report from an English hospital (Stern 1947). Although exclusive breastfeeding was entirely protective against diarrheal morbidity, mixed-feeding offered no protection to the English babies. The source of the illness was traced to contaminated bottles, which pose a persisent threat to children in resource-poor countries.

## Why Do Mothers Combine Feeding Methods?

The World Health Organization (1991:80) has noted that inadequate time has been dedicated to understanding why some women are resistant to breast-feeding. Why do most women in all countries supplement breastfeeding? Why do a few completely avoid breastfeeding? Frequently cited is the availability of formula, which certainly is a major factor. But women supplemented long before formula was invented, and the supplements they now use in resource-poor countries are often not formula. Many women feed inexpensive semi-solid foods, animal milks and canned products not made for babies. They mix sweetened cornstarch with water if that's all they can afford. If it looks "milky," it ends up in baby bottles. The idea of "natural" breastfeeding has been called a myth (Obermeyer and Castle 1997).

UNICEF described what happened in Barbados. Although bottles were banned and mothers were educated, they still did not breastfeed very much. UNICEF noted especially that women's employers and their male partners did not support them. UNICEF's Executive Director James Grant (1984:32) said, "It is no wonder that the mothers gave up."

The reasons why most women supplement are remarkably similar in all countries, industrialized or resource-poor. Many women are like those in Barbados in that they work away from their babies, in field and factory. Some mothers are so overworked that they find it difficult to allot the time to sit and breastfeed (Forman 1984). Family members and friends often suggest bottles or offer to feed the baby.

Even mothers who are with their babies all day often supplement. It is extremely common for women to believe that they do not have enough milk, even when they do. "Insufficient milk syndrome" is found in all regions of the world, among malnourished and well-nourished women. When babies cry for no apparent reason, breastfeeding women worry that they do not have enough milk. Women are often also afraid their milk is weak or does not agree with the baby. Mothers in Kenya were asked why almost all of them supplemented. They also said that they didn't always have enough milk or that their babies were either crying, hungry, teething or had stomach aches. They said that their husbands and relatives wanted to feed the baby (Mukuria 1996).

Mothers in Bogotá, Colombia, seemed to feel that preparing complex food mixtures for their babies was equated with greater care and love. They made elaborate soups to balance "hot" and "cold" elements rather than breastfeed. Van Esterik (1988:194) noted, "Clearly, in Bogotá, mothers do not realize the convenient, fast way to feed an infant."

Some mothers supplement their breastmilk because health workers tell them to. This is not limited to industrialized countries. Health workers in rural Malawi believed that the main problem with breastfeeding was "insufficient milk." In all cases, they recommended that mothers deal with the problem by supplementing (Castle 1993). The health workers could have told mothers to nurse more frequently to build up their milk supply, but they did not.

Mothers in Cairo, Egypt, believed that combining formula with breastfeeding increased the nutritional quality of the child's diet (National Control of Diarrheal Diseases Project 1988). As in most cultures, it was traditional for women to supplement breastfeeding with other liquids and semisolids. This often began in the first or second month of life, but may have begun hours after delivery.

Mothers in Honduras saw breastfeeding as a sacrifice. They knew that bottle-fed babies were sick more, but they weighed the increased risk of illnesses against convenience and the advantage of having a fat, undemanding baby (Cohen 1995b). They wanted other people to feed the baby, they wanted time away and they thought that their babies should get used to other foods.

Breastfeeding is extremely important and meaningful to some women (especially breastfeeding advocates). But to many poor women in resource-poor countries, breastfeeding is a "run-of-the-mill necessity and sometimes something that interferes with their chance to improve their days and better the lives of their children" (Raphael and Davis 1985). When breastfeeding becomes inconvenient for working mothers in Africa, Asia and Latin America, they may nurse only at night or stop breastfeeding altogether. Even women who do agricultural work may no longer be able to breastfeed during the day. Along with a push for African countries to pay off their debts to international lending agencies came changes in the agricultural patterns. Now there are more large tracts of land devoted to raising crops for export. This may have done a little good in paying off the enormous debts, but it certainly has not been good for breastfeeding. When women worked their own small plots of land for subsistence farming, they could stop and nurse their babies. But women who walk long distances to work on large agricultural tracts often leave their babies at home. In Zambia, formula feeding is considered a necessity for mothers who work outside the home (Geloo 1998).

In various cultures additional factors interfere with exclusive breastfeeding. Single fathers buy formula as a way of contributing to their child's upbringing (Ridler 1996). Bottle-feeding is so ingrained in Jamaica that women were undeterred by rising prices of formula (Melville 1991). The availability of baby sitters is another factor. Popkin (1978) reported that the number of daughters aged 13 to 15 in poor homes in the Philippines had a significant negative effect on the duration of breastfeeding.

Jelliffe and Jelliffe, whose lives were spent supporting breastfeeding in resource-poor countries, noted the reasons why mothers prefer mixed-feeding:

> Mixed feeding may be especially appealing to mothers, as an apparent doubling of nutritional protection and, in some communities, as a prepared insurance in case she wishes to work or find employment. The immediate risk of diarrhoeal disease and the interference with breast-milk production are not adequately appreciated. (1978:218)

Van Esterik (1989:176-177) noted,

> Just as the picture of a feeding bottle containing a marasmic infant has been a powerful symbol for the activists seeking to limit the promotion of infant formula in developing countries, so the feeding bottle for many women in the third world is a symbol of their freedom from worry about the quality and quantity of their milk.

Not only do breastfeeding mothers use bottles, bottle-feeding mothers sometimes offer the breast. Why? One reason is that the breast is seen in many cultures as a primary way to comfort a fussy baby. The German word for breastfeed is *stillen*, to make still or to quiet. In traditional societies, the breast is the way to soothe a baby. They do not use pacifiers (dummies), or baby swings, or tape recordings of sounds from the womb. Mothers in resource-poor countries who can afford to bottle-feed may do so when they're alone, but breastfeed in the presence of relatives who disapprove of bottle-feeding. A mother whose breasts are uncomfortably full after her milk comes in may suckle her baby.

Also significant is the fact that, in many cultures, mothers and babies sleep together, allowing the child to suckle when mothers are asleep. This is common in almost all cultures, although in some cultures cosleeping is frowned upon and kept secret. There are many stories from the United States — where many disapprove of cosleeping — of chubby "formula fed" babies who don't drink much formula. But they do sleep with their mothers. Since an HIV-positive, bottle-feeding mother offering her breast for any reason would expose her baby to the virus, some advise HIV-positive women not to cosleep, lest the babies take the breast while mothers are sleeping. Others advise HIV-positive mothers to cosleep to encourage bonding.

## Why Mixed Feeding Is Relatively Nonprotective

Breastfeeding researchers maintain that intestinal flora and the pH of the infant's gut render mixed-feeding nonprotective. Although water supplements can cause illness — if the water is contaminated — milk or food-based supplements have a negative impact even when they are clean and properly prepared. They don't cause illness directly, but they do change the intestinal flora and raise the gut pH, making it more alkaline. With higher gut pH, it is easier for undesirable microorganisms and gram-negative bacteria to take hold.

Exclusively breastfed babies have fecal flora in which healthy bacteria predominate (Chierici 1997), which is why exclusively breastfed babies have mild-smelling stools. But once breastfed babies are given supplements, other bacteria predominate. Additional foods or fluids alter the gut pH (Heinig & Dewey 1996). Although older studies (Bullen 1976, Dolby 1977) reported a greater difference in bacteria than do more recent studies (Balmer 1994, Kleesen 1995, Sepp 1997, Wold and Adlerberth 1998), babies in resource-poor countries are not generally fed modern, well-prepared formulas. When they are mixed-fed, their gut flora are not like that of exclusively breastfed babies (Bezirtzoglou and Romond 1989).

Years ago Bullen (1976) reported that the gut pH of "breastfed" babies who were given formula did not return to levels typical of breastfed babies until up to several weeks after supplementation ended. During times of more alkaline pH, which for mixed-fed babies is all the time, undesirable microorganisms can take hold. Researchers in Pakistan found that mixed-feeding (breast and bottle) was protective (Ashraf 1991), but most of the infants observed were supplemented with water only (Jalil 1990).

## The Hypothesis That Exclusive Breastfeeding Will Protect Against HIV Infection

It has been hypothesized that exclusive breastfeeding by an HIV-infected mother may be less likely to infect her infant than mixed-feeding (O'Gara and Martin 1996, Greiner 1997b). This is the premise: "NOTHING else must be given since almost anything may initiate bacterial, allergic or food intolerance processes that damage the immature gut and presumably increase the risk of transfer of HIV if it is present in the breast milk" (Greiner 1997b).

One difficulty in conceptualizing how to protect babies is that no one is clear about where infection via breastmilk happens. Gerold and Adler (1992) hypothesized that breastfeeding children may be infected at any point from their mouths to the glands in their anal sinuses. HIV infection may be more likely to happen in the mouth when babies have oral lesions. Or HIV can also infect babies when they have teeth erupting, as Langerhans cells (a type of dendritic cell which transports antigens to the lymph nodes) are heavily concentrated within fissures between babies' teeth. Also, the areola (the darker area around the nipple) is supplied with lymphatic vessels; if babies bite at the nipple/areola, lymph vessels may burst and lymph, which contains infected T-cells, can infect the baby's epithelium. Gerold and Adler also pointed out that the desirable low pH in a baby's gastrointestinal tract is not present at birth but decreases gradually. Immediately after birth, the baby's stomach pH is 7.4, which is not low enough to inactivate HIV, regardless of how carefully the newborn is treated. HIV could then infect the Langerhans cells of the stomach, duodenum, colon or rectum. As it reaches the anal canal in fecal matter, it can enter the glands in the anal sinuses.

## Clarifying Breastfeeding Styles

The idea that exclusively breastfeeding would be less likely to transmit the virus is still a hypothesis. Tess (1997) found that Brazilian babies who were fed only breastmilk and water were less likely to become HIV-infected than babies who were fed breastmilk plus other foods. But two other studies found that exclusive breastfeeding by HIV-infected mothers was associated with higher rates of HIV infection. Ryder and colleagues (1991) examined patterns of morbidity in a report about HIV-1 infection in Zaire. Two-thirds of the mothers had chosen to combine breast and bottle-feeding. Their 68 mixed-fed infants were referred to as "not breastfed" and, for analysis of morbidity, were combined with the 10 infants who were exclusively bottle-fed, rather than with the 28 who were exclusively breastfed. It is not at all clear why most researchers have failed to differentiate babies according to how they are fed (breast, bottle and mixed).

Ryder found that exclusively breastfed babies actually had a very slightly higher rate of infection (20 percent) than the mixed-fed babies, only 19 percent of whom were infected. (The rate of transmission for the exclusively bottle-fed infants was zero percent.) Ryder also noted that the rates of morbidity were significantly higher for children who were "not breastfed," which is the term he used to describe both bottle-fed and mixed-fed babies.

Bobat and colleagues (1997) in South Africa also reported that exclusively breastfed babies had a higher rate of HIV transmission than mixed-fed babies. Thirty-nine percent of the exclusively breastfed babies became HIV-infected, compared to 32 percent of the mixed-fed babies and 24 percent of the formula-fed babies. The longer babies were exclusively breastfed, the greater the risk of HIV infection. Among babies exclusively breastfed for one month, 45 percent became HIV-infected. Of babies exclusively breastfed for two months, the rate of infection climbed to 64 percent, and babies exclusively breastfed for three months stood an alarming 75 percent chance of becoming HIV-infected.

It has also been suggested that exclusively breastfed babies also need to be spared all intrusive procedures during birth, as these might open a portal for infection. There is no research that looked specifically at combining exclusivity with protection from invasive procedures. Nevertheless, health care workers in endemic areas now try to spare babies from any procedure that might increase the risk of infection before or during birth.

## How Doable Is a Return to Exclusivity Now?

Given the enormous benefits of exclusive breastfeeding for babies of non-infected mothers (the vast majority), it is understandable that UNICEF, the WHO and other groups have put great efforts into trying to restore exclusivity. The earliest such campaigns had not succeeded in Trinidad (Gueri 1978), Costa Rica (Mata 1983), South Africa (Ross 1983), Barbados (Grant 1986), or Indonesia (Zeitlin 1984). Later interventions also failed to restore exclusivity. Greiner (1993) referred to these two statements as fibs: "Yes, we know why breastfeeding is declining" and "Yes, we know what to do about it."

Koctürk and Zetterström (1988) pointed out that it is difficult to promote breastfeeding when women feel that it prevents them from improving their socioeconomic status. Despite the work of the past two decades, family members, friends and even health care systems still discourage exclusive breastfeeding (Lutter 1996). David and David (1984) reported from Yemen, "The militant stance against the bottle on the part of the health center's staff did not prevent widespread bottle feeding." It is still easier to achieve a change from no breastfeeding to partial breastfeeding than it is to achieve a change from partial breastfeeding to exclusive breastfeeding (Dimond and Ashworth 1987).

The most recent attempts to restore exclusivity have been quite labor-intensive, and so are relevant to discussions about any kind of infant-feeding teaching. It has been suggested that studies about replacement feeding would not yield replicable results because the HIV-positive mothers in the studies would be taught how to safely formula-feed. That is likely to be true. But then again, some programs in the last two decades have gone to enormous lengths to teach exclusive breastfeeding.

Cohen (1995a) reported that she and colleagues wanted to study the growth patterns of exclusively breastfed infants in Honduras. They maintained exclusivity by hospitalizing women three times for a three-day stay in the "La Leche League unit" of the hospital. In addition, these women were visited weekly to maintain exclusive breastfeeding. Women who began solids or liquids were counseled to stop. Even so, some women admitted to supplementing breastfeeding. They were dropped from the study. Of the 453 women who agreed to the study design, were hospitalized for three three-day stays in the La Leche unit, and who were then visited weekly for the sole purpose of maintaining exclusive breastfeeding, only 164 were compliant by the sixteenth week.

In the Islamic Republic of Iran, UNICEF collaborated with the Ministry of Health, the religious leaders, and the universities and nongovernmental organizations to undertake a massive breastfeeding campaign. In theory, breastfeeding promotion should not have been necessary, as the Koran advocates two years of breastfeeding. (The Islamic Republic of Iran is a Moslem theocracy that follows the Koran.) But the breastfeeding campaign was seen as necessary and was welcomed by Iranian public health officials (Saadeh 1993). There was face-to-face communication during the Imams' Friday prayers. A primary health care staff was trained and sent to do door-to-door canvassing and to make additional contacts. In addition to the door-to-door contacts, there was a very active media campaign, with broadcasts at prime time. There were breastfeeding comedies with famous actors, breastfeeding children's programs and breastfeeding quizzes and literacy programs. The government of Iran banned the sale of formula without a prescription. But a black market situation broke out, which allowed citizens to obtain formula without a prescription. Although many women did breastfeed, some Iranian women were still resistant, buying black market formula instead.

Women's fondness for formula was the subject of a report about a brand manufactured in Switzerland, sold to Uzbekistan, and then smuggled to other Central Asian Republics, Iran and Pakistan (IBFAN 1998:40). Women in Kenya said that the only reason why they didn't use formula was that they couldn't afford it (Latham 1988:92). Health workers in Rwanda said that the reason why they didn't need to promote breastfeeding was that most people couldn't afford formula (Wellstart 1994).

Monteiro and colleagues (1990) reported from Brazil that "ambitious" efforts had been able to extend the duration of exclusive breastfeeding from just under one month to two months. The ambitious efforts involved intensive use of mass media, training of health care workers and reorganization of the routine activities of the health services. While breastfeeding prevalence in Brazil rose by 20 percent after the extensive campaign, prevalence "dropped back almost to pre-campaign levels after the program was suspended in 1985" (USAID 1990:45).

A program on the outskirts of Mexico City was quite effective in maintaining exclusive breastfeeding, but it required one-to-one home visits (Morrow 1996). The program trained lay breastfeeding counselors and sent them into mothers' homes to encourage exclusive breastfeeding. Among the group that did not receive any home visits, only 7 percent of the mothers practiced exclusive breastfeeding. Among the mothers who received six home visits, 48 percent practiced exclusive breastfeeding. Many of these mothers did give some supplements, but stopped after being visited again.

Haider's report from Bangladesh (1996a, 1996b) clarified that the "exclusively breastfed" hospitalized babies were really being mixed-fed. Haider cured the babies' diarrhea by providing counselors to teach the mothers to switch from mixed-feeding to exclusive breastfeeding. But without one-to-one counseling, many mothers failed to continue breastfeeding exclusively even after their babies had been discharged from the hospital.

## A Study That Has Been Used to Suggest That Lack of BreastFeeding Is Almost Always Fatal

One report has been cited to dramatize the dangers of nonbreastfeeding. Scrimshaw's 1968 study of seven Punjab villages in India reported a first-year death rate of 950 per 1000 for infants artificially fed at birth. But these babies were not bottle-fed formula. The infants who could feed at all sucked on cloth or cotton wool dipped into brass bowls containing sugar or honey water, or highly diluted goat, buffalo or cow milk. The water diluting the milks was not boiled, and the bowls sat under beds until the contents were exhausted.

Scrimshaw observed 20 nonbreastfed babies, ten of whom were too weak or premature to suck. It is not surprising that 19 of the 20 died, more than half in the first week and another four by one month. Two babies who died had mothers who were dead, and another had a gravely ill mother. Mortality rates for orphaned babies in such settings are traditionally high. Two mothers had no milk, and five babies would not take the breast. Yet a later report about Scrimshaw's work gives a different impression:

> The infant-mortality rate in the artificially fed was 950 per 1000 live births compared with 120 in the breast-fed. Differences were in large measure due to diarrhoeal disease and malnutrition, but also include other conditions, such as respiratory-tract infections, whose effects are often underestimated. (Jelliffe and Jelliffe 1978:289)

The above analysis, however, would have been more accurate if it had noted that many of the babies were too weak or premature to suck and died in the first week. Furthermore, the report would have been more accurate if it noted that even the youngest babies were sucking small amounts of overdiluted unclean fluids from cotton wool or cloths out of bowls that sat under beds. Teapot-like vessels were also used for babies. Some older babies sipped liquids from little cups or were fed from any kind of bottle with a nipple attached. Scrimshaw's report on the cotton wool/cloth/teapot-fed babies does not prove that babies bottle-fed formula die at a rate of 950 out of 1000.

## Studies That Are Not Cited

While a few studies are cited in discussions about HIV and infant feeding, more are omitted. The following studies have reported the same two findings, that exclusive breastfeeding is uncommon and that supplemented breastfeeding is relatively nonprotective: Brown 1989, Clemens 1997, David and David 1984, Grantham-McGregor 1970, Gurwith 1983, Haider 1996b, López-Alarcón 1997, Mondal 1996, Plank and Milanesi 1973, Popkin 1990, Vis 1981, Zohoori 1993. These studies argue strongly against the assertion that a switch from the current pattern (mixed-feeding) to nonbreastfeeding would result in higher mortality rates than one finds among babies breastfed by HIV-infected mothers.

Breastfeeding just looks best when there is no talk about the mediocre benefits of mixed-feeding. In an HIV analysis of a hypothetical resource-poor country in East Africa, the possible effects of mixed-feeding were "not considered," although it was noted that any switch to mixed-feeding "would be entirely deleterious" (Del Fante 1993). Another analysis about HIV and breastfeeding compared infants entirely denied the breast with "optimally breastfed infants" (Kuhn and Stein 1997).

## How Much Does Breastfeeding (or Mixed-Feeding) Reduce Mortality?

Citing numerous studies (Grant 1985, 1986, 1987), UNICEF had long warned that bottle-feeding doubled or tripled infant mortality. From UNICEF's 1986 *State of the World's Children* report came a statement comparing the two extremes, of exclusive bottle-feeding and exclusive breastfeeding: "In dozens of surveys in poor communities, it has now been shown that bottle-fed babies are as much as *two or three times* as likely to die in infancy than babies who are exclusively breast-fed for the first few months" (Grant 1986:55–56).

UNICEF's 1990 *State of the World's Children* report made the point that breastfeeding's early protection is significantly weakened by supplements: "In those early months, even supplementing breast-feeding with powdered milk can bring a ten-fold increase in the risk of death" (Grant 1990:26).

The point of the first UNICEF statement is that a switch from exclusive breastfeeding to exclusive bottle-feeding doubles or triples risks. The second statement asserts that mixed-feeding increases mortality rates tenfold over exclusive breastfeeding. Considered together (and taken with all the research), these two statements pack a powerful message. If a switch from exclusive breastfeeding doubles or triples mortality, then a switch from (one-tenth-as-good) mixed-feeding may not even double mortality.

## HIV Analyses That Acknowledge Neither the Pervasiveness Nor the Mediocrity of Mixed-Feeding

In this era, when breastfeeding seems threatened by HIV, breastfeeding's benefits are being very strongly defended. Many HIV analyses do not tell readers that most "breastfeeding" today is really mixed-feeding, or that mixed-feeding offers mediocre health benefits. Many HIV analyses do not inform readers that the major switch will be from mediocre mixed-feeding (not exclusive breastfeeding) to nonbreastfeeding. New HIV discussions give the impression that a switch from any breastfeeding would increase mortality fourteenfold: "Death from diarrhea is 14 times higher in artificially fed infants than in those who are breastfed" (Bellamy 1998:30).

The statistics on exclusive breastfeeding versus exclusive bottle-feeding from the diarrhea section of one study in Brazil (Victora 1987) make dramatic reading. But it is time to acknowledge the mortality risks of actual feeding patterns, and to factor into HIV risk-benefit analyses information about the mediocre benefits of mixed-feeding. It is also time to consider other research studies, in addition to the few favorable breastfeeding studies that are cited over and over again.

## AIDS-Generated Avoidance of Breastfeeding

The traditional breastfeeding literature argues that Third World babies would suffer from greatly increased mortality and morbidity if they were not breastfed. But the few results available to date suggest that this is not necessarily the case in some settings, especially where mothers are taught how to carry out safe replacement feeding. Gray's research, for instance, reported in 1996 and 1997 that breastfed babies in Soweto, South Africa, were twice as likely to become HIV-infected as bottle-fed babies. This finding corroborates earlier breast-versus-bottle reports from France (Blanche 1989), Italy (Gabiano 1992), Australia (Dunn 1992) and Zaire (Ryder 1991). But Gray also reported that the bottle-fed babies were just as healthy as the breastfed babies. There was neither an increased risk of gastro-intestinal or respiratory infections nor a greater occurrence of hospital admissions. Growth patterns were equivalent. The Soweto group (Urban 1997) also reported that 2 out of 100 HIV-positive mothers had problems bonding emotionally with their babies. Women with an infectious terminal disease, who are worried about harming their babies, might be expected to have problems bonding. But the two Soweto women were both breastfeeding mothers. No bottle-feeding mothers were noted to have problems in bonding (Urban 1997).

Bobat's report from Durban, South Africa, called into question another traditional belief — that exclusively breastfed babies always do better than bottle-fed or mixed-fed babies. Mortality, which occurred only among HIV-infected infants, was highest among those who were exclusively breastfed, with a 19 percent mortality rate. Among the mixed-fed, mortality was 13 percent; among the formula-fed, zero percent. There was no difference between the three groups in the frequency of non-HIV-related complications like diarrhea, respiratory infections and problems with growth. Bobat (1997) suggested HIV-positive women "should be advised that breastfeeding may not provide the anticipated degree of protection against common infections and growth failure, and is associated with a higher risk of transmission."

Why were Gray's bottle-fed babies just as healthy as her breastfed babies? Perhaps because her "breastfed" babies were not exclusively breastfed but were given semisolid foods even at an early age. Why did Bobat's exclusively breastfed babies have so many problems and the highest mortality rates? Perhaps because the milk of immunocompromised HIV-infected women has lesser amounts of protective factors, an issue that needs study.

Perhaps the availability of clean water in South Africa contributed to the relative safety of formula feeding. Some mothers had clean water at home, and other mothers obtained water from a community tap. Also significant is the fact that mothers were taught how to safely prepare clean bottles of formula (Urban 1997). All of these factors are likely to contribute to the relative safety of replacement feeding.

## Safe and Not-So-Safe Replacement Feeding

A report from Bombay, India, gave clear evidence of the dangers of unsupported bottle-feeding in a resource-poor country (Damania 1998). Of 320 HIV-positive women, 59 chose the avoidance of breastfeeding as their only intervention, opting not to receive AZT and not to have a cesarean delivery. Of these 59 nonbreastfeeding mother-baby pairs, two babies died of infective gastroenteritis related to bottle-feeding. An additional three babies were hospitalized with diarrhea but responded to treatment.

Clearly it is not enough to recommend that HIV-positive mothers avoid breastfeeding. They need support in learning how to make replacement feeding as safe as possible. Otherwise, there will be little point in advising them to consider not breastfeeding. In a document prepared for a World Health Organization Technical Consultation, Dr. Ruth Nduati (1998) stated that replacement feeding should be "supported with health education on safe handling." Mothers in Nduati's Nairobi cohort teach one another how to formula feed safely and usually feed formula in cups. The children of the HIV-positive women in this cohort do very well with the extra attention they receive.

HIV-positive mothers in Brazil have also been able to safely bottle-feed formula with the benefit of teaching (Rubini 1994). Shaffer (1998) noted that HIV-positive new mothers in Thailand are taught how to formula feed safely during their two-day stays in the hospital. They are also followed up with extensive counseling to be sure that they are not breastfeeding and that they are formula-feeding safely. The government of Botswana is considering ways to support HIV-positive mothers interested in formula-feeding (Anabwani 1998).

The idea of teaching mothers how to carry out safe replacement-feeding seems to be at odds with the major goal of restoring exclusive breastfeeding, but years ago health workers who became pessimistic about restoring breastfeeding in Yemen had taught mothers how to bottle-feed (Greiner 1997a).

## Partial Prolonged Breastfeeding

In decades of trying, UNICEF, the WHO and other groups have not been able to convince most women to breastfeed exclusively. This is not surprising since societies have not lightened the burdens that keep women from breastfeeding exclusively. The common pattern of partial breastfeeding often continues for many months, sometimes into the second or third year of life, and occasionally longer. Forty-seven percent of children in sub–Saharan Africa are still breastfeeding at age 20-23 months, as are 65 percent in South Asia and 67 percent in India (Bellamy 1998).

If one were to imagine the worst feeding pattern for the child of an

HIV-infected mother, it would be partial prolonged breastfeeding. In the early months the result is mediocre health, which is followed by the increasing risk of HIV transmission as the partial breastfeeding continues. Even for children of initially HIV-negative mothers, this feeding practice poses some risk. HIV-negative mothers who become newly infected while breastfeeding risk infecting their breastfeeding children. Given the low rates of testing, it is likely that a large percentage of the HIV-infected mothers on earth are practicing partial prolonged breastfeeding — the worst possible option.

---

# References

Acheson, E. D., and S. C. Truelove. 1961. Early weaning in the aetiology of ulcerative colitis. *British Medical Journal* ii: 929–931.

*Affordable Options for the Prevention of Mother-to-Child Transmission of HIV-1.* 1997. Johannesburg, South Africa, November 19–20. National AIDS Programme and the Perinatal HIV Research Unit.

Akré, J., ed. 1989. Infant feeding: The physiological basis. *Bulletin of the World Health Organization*, supplement to Vol. 67.

al-Mazroui, M. J., C. O. Oyejide, A. Bener and M. Y. Cheema. 1997. Breastfeeding and supplemental feeding for neonates in Al-Ain, United Arab Emirates. *Journal of Tropical Pediatrics* 43: 304–306.

American Academy of Pediatrics Work Group in Breastfeeding. 1997. Breastfeeding and the use of human milk. *Pediatrics* 100: 1035–1039.

Anabwani, Gabriel. 1998. Panel on clinical management and biomedical advances of the Satellite Meeting of the Harvard AIDS Institute, Twelfth World AIDS Conference, Geneva, Switzerland, June 27.

Arnon, S. S. 1986. Infant botulism: Anticipating the second decade. *Journal of Infectious Diseases* 154: 201–206.

Ashraf, Rifat Nisar, et al. 1991. Breast-feeding and protection against neonatal sepsis in high risk population. *Archives of Disease in Childhood* 66: 488–490.

Azaiza, Feisal. 1995. Patterns of breastfeeding among rural Moslem women in Israel: A descriptive account. *Israel Journal of Medical Science* 31: 411–417.

Balmer, S. E., and B. A. Wharton. 1991. Diet and faecal flora in the newborn: Iron. *Archives of Disease in Childhood* 66: 1390–1394.

Balmer, S. E., L. S. Hanvey and B. A. Wharton. 1994. Diet and faecal flora in the newborn: Nucleotides. *Archives of Disease in Childhood* 70: F137–F140.

Barrington-Ward, S. 1997. *The Progress of Nations 1997: Nutrition Commentary.* New York: UNICEF.

Bellamy, Carol. 1998. *The State of the World's Children.* New York: UNICEF.

Bezirtzoglou, Eugenia, and Charles Romond. 1989. Effect of the feeding practices on the establishment of bacterial interactions in the intestine of the newborn delivered by cesarean section. *Journal of Perinatal Medicine* 17: 139–143.

Blanche, S., et al. 1989. A prospective study of perinatal infection of infants born to women seropositive for human immunodeficiency virus type 1. *New England Journal of Medicine* 320: 1643–1648.

Bobat, R., Moodley Dhayendree, Anna Coutsoudis and Hoosen Coovadia. 1997. Breastfeeding by HIV-1-infected women and outcome in their infants: A cohort study from Durban, South Africa. *AIDS* 11: 1627–1633.

Boerma, J. T., et al. 1991. Bottle use for infant feeding in resource-poor countries: Data from the Demographic and Health Surveys. Has the bottle battle been lost? *Journal of Tropical Pediatrics* 37: 116–120.

Brennemann, J. 1923. Artificial feeding of infants. In *Pediatrics*, ed. I. A. Abt. Philadelphia: W. B. Saunders Company.

Brown, K. H., R. E. Black, G. Lopez de Romana and H. Creed de Kanashiro. 1989. Infant-feeding practices and their relationship with diarrhoeal and other diseases in Huascar (Lima), Peru. *Pediatrics* 83: 31–44.

Bullen, C. L., P. V. Tearle and A. T. Willis. 1976. Bifidobacteria in the intestinal tract of infants – an in vivo study. *Journal of Medical Microbiology* 9: 325–333.

Cantrelle, P., and H. Leridon. 1971. Mortality in childhood and fertility in a rural zone of Senegal. *Population Studies* 25: 505–533.

Carter, Pam. 1995. *Feminism, Breasts and Breast-Feeding.* New York: St. Martin's Press.

Castle, Sarah E. 1993. *The Social Context of Breastfeeding and Early Supplementation in Chikwawa District, Malawi.* A report to Wellstart and the International Eye Foundation, Washington, D.C.

Chierici, R., et al. 1997. Experimental milk formulae with reduced protein content and desialylated milk proteins: Influence on the faecal flora and the growth of term newborn infants. *Acta Paediatrica Supplement* 86: 557–563.

Clavanno, N. R. 1982. Mode of feeding and its effect on infant mortality and morbidity. *Journal of Tropical Pediatrics* 28: 287–293.

Clemens, John D., et al. 1993. Breast-feeding and the risk of life-threatening rotavirus diarrhea: Prevention or postponement? *Pediatrics* 92: 680–685.

_____. 1997. 1. Breastfeeding and the risk of life-threatening enterotoxigenic escherichia coli diarrhea in Bangladeshi infants and children. *Pediatrics* 100 (6), December: e2.

Cohen, R. J., et al. 1995a. Determinants of growth from birth to 12 months among breast-fed Honduran infants in relation to age of introduction of complementary foods. *Pediatrics* 96: 504–510.

_____. 1995b. Maternal activity budgets: Feasibility of exclusive breastfeeding for six months among urban women in Honduras. *Social Science and Medicine* 41: 527–536.

Coreil, Jeannine, et al. 1998. Cultural feasibility studies in preparation for clinical trials to reduce maternal-infant HIV transmission in Haiti. *AIDS Education and Prevention* 10: 46–62.

Cunningham, Allan S., Derrick B. Jelliffe, E. F. Patrice Jelliffe. 1991. Breast-feeding and health in the 1980s: A global epidemiologic review. *Journal of Pediatrics* 118: 659–666.

Cunningham, Allan S. 1995. Breastfeeding: Adaptive behavior for child health and longevity. In *Breastfeeding Biocultural Perspectives*, eds. Patricia Stuart-Macadam and Katherine A. Dettwyler. New York: Aldine De Gruyter, pp. 243–264.

Damania, Kaizad, et al. 1998. Three pronged strategy to prevent mother to child transmission. Presented at the Twelfth World AIDS Conference, Geneva, Switzerland, June 28–July 3. Abstract 23324.

David, C. B., and P. H. David. 1984. Bottle-feeding and malnutrition in a resource-poor country: The "bottle-starved" baby. *Journal of Tropical Pediatrics* 30: 159–164.

Davis, Margaret, D. A. Savitz and B. I. Graubard. 1988. Infant feeding and childhood cancer. *Lancet* 2: 365–368.

Del Fante, P., et al. 1993. HIV, breast-feeding & under-5 mortality: Modeling the impact of policy decisions for or against breast-feeding. *Journal of Tropical Medicine and Hygiene* 96: 203–211.

Dimond, Hilary J., and Ann Ashworth. 1987. Infant feeding practices in Kenya, Mexico and Malaysia: The rarity of the exclusively breastfed infant. *Human Nutrition: Applied Nutrition* 41A: 51–64.

Division of Child Health and Development, World Health Organization. 1998. *Improving Child Health: The Integrated Approach*. Geneva, Switzerland: World Health Organization.

Dolby, J. M., P. Honour and H. B. Valman. 1977. Bacteriostasis of E. coli by milk. I. Colonization of breastfed infants by milk resistant organisms. *Journal of Hygiene* 78: 85–94.

Dugdale, A. E. 1971. The effect of the type of feeding on weight gain and illnesses in infants. *British Journal of Nutrition* 26: 423–432.

Duncan, B. J. Ey, et al. 1993. Exclusive breast-feeding for at least 4 months protects against otitis media. *Pediatrics* 91: 867–872.

Dunn, D. T., M.-L. Newell, A. E. Ades, C. S. Peckham. 1992. Risk of human immunodeficiency virus type 1 transmission through breastfeeding. *Lancet* 340: 585–588.

Feachem, R. G., and M. A. Koblinsky. 1984. Interventions for the control of diarrheal disease among young children: Promotion of breastfeeding. *Bulletin of the World Health Organization* 62: 271–291.

Forman, Michele R. 1984. Review of research on the factors associated with choice and duration of infant feeding in less-developed countries. *Pediatrics Supplement* 667: 667–694.

Gabiano, Clara, et al. 1992. Mother-to-child transmission of HIV type 1: Risk of infection and correlates of transmission. *Pediatrics* 90: 69–74.

Geloo, Zarina. 1998. HIV and breastfeeding: Reigniting an old controversy. Women's Feature Service. *Women's International Net Magazine*. Available at http://www. geocities.com/wellesley/3321/win6d.htm; INTERNET.

Gerold, M., and R. Adler. 1992. Manifestations of pediatric AIDS: Proposed mechanisms of transmission. *Medical Hypotheses* 37: 205–212.

Glass, Roger I., et al. 1986. Questions concerning a protective role for breast-feeding in severe rotavirus diarrhea. *Acta Paediatrica* 75: 713–718.

Grant, James P. 1984. *The State of the World's Children*. New York: UNICEF.

_____. 1985. *The State of the World's Children*. New York: UNICEF.

_____. 1986. *The State of the World's Children*. New York: UNICEF.

_____. 1987. *The State of the World's Children*. New York: UNICEF.

_____. 1990. *The State of the World's Children*. New York: UNICEF.

Grantham-McGregor, S. M., and E. H. Black. 1970. Breast feeding in Kingston, Jamaica. *Archives of Disease in Childhood* 45: 404–409.

Gray, Glenda, J. A. McIntyre and S. F. Lyons. 1996. The effect of breastfeeding on vertical transmission of HIV-1 in Soweto, South Africa. Presented at the Eleventh International Conference on AIDS, Vancouver, Canada, July 7–12. Abstract Th.C.415.

Gray, Glenda E. 1997. Breastfeeding-related transmission. Presented at the Fourth International Conference on AIDS in Asia and the Pacific, Manila, Philippines, October 25–29. Abstract FA10.

Greco, L., S. Auricchio, M. Mayer and M. Grimaldi. 1988. Case control study on nutritional risk factors in celiac disease. *Journal of Pediatric Gastroenterology and Nutrition* 7: 395–399.

Greiner, Ted. 1983. The planning, implementation and evaluation of a project to protect, support and promote breastfeeding in the Yemen Arab Republic, Ph.D. dissertation, Cornell University, Ithaca, New York.

_____. 1993. Breastfeeding communication strategies, adapted from *Infant and Young Child Nutrition: A Historic Review from a Communication Perspective*. Introduction to *Communication Strategies to Support Infant and Young Child Nutrition*, ed. Peggy Kojniz-Booher. Cornell University Monographs 24–25, pp. 7–15.

_____. 1997a. Breastfeeding and LAM: Beyond conventional approaches. Modified from paper presented at the Georgetown University Institute for Reproductive Health End of Project Conference "Bellagio and Beyond," Washington, D.C., May 15–16.

_____. 1997b. The HIV threat to breastfeeding: Virus, fear and greed. Modified from a talk to the Bangladeshi Breastfeeding Foundation, August 29.

Gueri, M., P. Jutsum and A. White. 1978. Evaluation of a breast-feeding campaign in Trinidad. *Bulletin of the Pan American Health Organization* 12: 112–115.

Gurwith, M., et al. 1983. Diarrhea among infants and young children in Canada: A longitudinal study in three Northern communities. *Journal of Infectious Diseases* 147: 685–692.

Habicht, Jean-Pierre, Julie Da Vanzo and William P. Butz. 1986. Does breastfeeding really save lives or are apparent benefits due to biases? *American Journal of Epidemiology* 123(2): 279–290.

Haider, R., et al. 1996a. Breast-feeding counseling in a diarrheal disease hospital. *Bulletin of the World Health Organization* 74: 173–179.

Haider, R., A. Islam, I. Kabir and D. Habte. 1996b. Early complementary feeding is associated with low nutritional status of young infants recovering from diarrhoea. *Journal of Tropical Pediatrics* 42: 170–172.

Hanson, L. A., et al. 1986. Breastfeeding in Reality. In *Human Lactation* 2, eds. M. Hamosh and A. Goldman. New York: Plenum, pp. 1–12.

Harrison, Gail G., Sahar S. Zaghloul, Osman M. Galal and Azza Gabr. 1993. Breastfeeding and weaning in a poor urban neighborhood in Cairo, Egypt: Maternal beliefs and perceptions. *Social Science and Medicine* 36: 1063–1069.

Heinig, M. Jane, and Kathryn Dewey. 1996. Health advantages of breast feeding for infants: A critical review. *Nutrition Research Reviews* 9: 89–110.

Herrera, M. G., J. O. Moore, B. DeParesdes and M. Wagner. 1980. Maternal weight/ height and the effect of food supplementation during pregnancy and lactation. In *Maternal Nutrition During Pregnancy and Lactation: An Overview*, eds. H. Aebi and R. G. Whitehead. Bern: Hans Huber, pp. 213–227.

Hobcraft J. N., J. W. McDonald and S. O. Rutstein. 1985. Demographic determinants of infant and early child mortality: A comparative analysis. *Population Studies* 39: 363–385.

Humphrey, J. 1996. Report to Johns Hopkins School of Hygiene and Public Health about attendance at Workshop on Breast-feeding Choices for the HIV Seropositive Mother, Durban, South Africa, May 20–21.

International Baby Food Action Network, Penang. 1998. *Breaking the Rules, Stretching the Rules*. Penang, Malaysia: IBFAN Penang.

Ibrahim, M. M., L. A. Persson, M. M. Omar and S. Wall. 1992. Breast feeding and the dietary habits of children in rural Somalia. *Acta Paediatrica* 81: 480–483.

Jalil, F., et. al. 1990. Methodological problems in assessment of long-term health outcomes in breast-fed versus bottle-fed infants. In *Breastfeeding, Nutrition and Infant Growth in Developed and Emerging Countries*, eds. S. A. Atkison, L. A. Hanson and R. K. Chandra. St. John's, Newfoundland: ARTS Biomedical Publishers and Distributors, pp. 381–394.

Jelliffe, Derrick B., and E. F. Patrice Jelliffe. 1978. *Human Milk in the Modern World*. London: Oxford University Press.

Kahn, James. 1997. Infant feeding for HIV-infected mothers: Which strategies minimize mortality risk in different epidemiologic settings? Presented at the Conference on Global Strategies for the Prevention of HIV Transmission from Mothers to Infants, Washington, D.C., September 3–6.

Karjalainen, J., et al. 1992. A bovine albumin peptide as a possible trigger of insulin dependent diabetes mellitus. *New England Journal of Medicine* 327: 302–307.

Kero, P., and P. Piekkala. 1987. Factors affecting the occurrence of acute otitis media during the first year of life. *Acta Paediatrica Scandanavia* 76: 618–623.

Kleesen, B., H. Bunke, K. Tovar, et al. 1995. Influence of two infant formulas and human milk on the development of the faecal flora in newborn infants. *Acta Paediatrica* 84: 1347–1356.

Koletzko, S., et al. 1989. Role of infant feeding practices in development of Crohn's disease in childhood. *British Medical Journal* 299: 1617–1618.

Koctürk, T., and R. Zetterström. 1988. Breast-feeding and its promotion. *Acta Paediatrica Scandanavia* 77: 183–190.

Kuhn, Louise, and Zena Stein. 1997. Infant survival, HIV infection, and feeding alternatives in less-developed countries. *American Journal of Public Health* 87: 926–931.

Labbok, Miriam, and Katherine Krasovec. 1990. Toward consistency in breast-feeding definitions. *Studies in Family Planning* 21: 226–230.

Labbok, Miriam H., Mark Belsey and C. Jared Coffin. 1997. A call for consistency in defining breast-feeding. *American Journal of Public Health* 87(6): 1060–1061.

Lanner, L. J., J. P. Habicht and S. Kardjati. 1990. Breastfeeding protects infants in Indonesia against illness and weight loss due to illness. *American Journal of Epidemiology* 13: 322–331.

Latham, Michael C., et al. 1986. Infant feeding in urban Kenya: A pattern of early triple nipple feeding. *Journal of Tropical Pediatrics* 32: 276–280.

Latham, Michael C., K. Okoth Agunda and Terry Elliot. 1988. Infant feeding in Nairobi, Kenya. In *Feeding Infants in Four Societies*, eds. Beverly Winikoff, Mary Ann Castle and Virginia Hight Laukaran. New York: Greenwood Press, pp. 67–94.

Latham, Michael C., and Stina Almroth. 1996. *A Breastfeeding Culture Without Exclusive Breastfeeding in Lesotho*. Washington, D.C.: USAID.

Lawrence, Ruth A. 1994. *Breastfeeding: A Guide for the Medical Profession* (4th ed.). St. Louis: C. V. Mosby Company.

Lepage, P., C. Munyakazi and P. Hennart 1981. Breastfeeding and hospital mortality in children in Rwanda. *Lancet* ii: 409–411.

López-Alarcón, Mardya, Salvador Villalpando and Arturo Fajardo. 1997. Breast-feeding lowers the frequency and duration of acute respiratory infection and diarrhea in infants under six months of age. *Journal of Nutrition* 127: 436–443.

Lutter, Chessa. 1996. *Exclusive Breastfeeding Promotion: A Summary of Findings from EPB's Applied Research Program (1992–1996)*. Washington, D.C.: USAID.

Mata, L., et al. 1983. Promotion of breast-feeding, health and growth among hospital-born neonates and among infants of a rural area of Costa Rica. In *Diarrhea and Malnutrition: Interactions, Mechanisms and Interventions*, eds. L. C. Chen and N. S. Scrimshaw. New York: Plenum Press, pp. 177-202.

Melville, Bendley Fitzgerald. 1991. Breast feeding decline in changing socio-economic conditions: The case of Jamaica, 1983-1989 (letter). *Journal of Tropical Pediatrics* 37: 93–94.

Merrett, T. G., et al. 1988. Infant feeding and allergy: Twelve-month prospective study of 500 babies born in allergic families. *Annals of Allergy* 61: 13–20.

McLaren, D. S. 1966. An early account of infant feeding practices and malnutrition in east Africa. *Journal of Tropical Pediatrics* 12: 50–52.

Moller, M. S. G. 1961. Custom, pregnancy and child rearing in Tanganyika. *African Child Health*, September: 66-80.

Mondal, S. K., et al. 1996. Occurrence of diarrhoeal diseases in relation to infant feeding practices in a rural community in West Bengal, India. *Acta Paediatrica* 85: 1159–1162.

Monteiro, C., M. Rea and C. V. Victora. 1990. Can infant mortality be reduced by promoting breastfeeding? Evidence from São Paulo City. *Health Policy and Planning* 5: 23–29.

Morrow, Ardythe L., et al. 1996. The effectiveness of home-based counseling to promote exclusive breastfeeding among Mexican mothers. In *Exclusive Breastfeeding Promotion: A Summary of Findings from EPB's Applied Research Program (1992–1996)*. Washington, D.C.: USAID.

Mukuria, Altrena G., et al. 1996. Early complementary feeding: the role of social support networks. In *Exclusive Breastfeeding Promotion: A Summary of Findings from EPB's Applied Research Program (1992–1996)*. Washington, D.C.: USAID.

National Control of Diarrheal Diseases Project. 1988. Impact of the National Control of Diarrheal Diseases Project on infant and child mortality in Dakahilia, Egypt. *Lancet*, July 16: 145–148.

Nduati, Ruth. 1998. *HIV and Infant Feeding: A Review of HIV Transmission Through Breastfeeding*. UNICEF/UNAIDS/WHO.

Nicoll, A., J. Z. J. Killewo and C. Mgone. 1990. HIV and infant feeding practices: Epidemiological implications for sub–Saharan African countries. *AIDS* 4: 661–665.

Nurture and Institute for Reproductive Health. 1996. *Breastfeeding Saves Lives*. USAID.

Nutrition Division of the Uganda Ministry of Health, Child Health and Development Center of Makerere University and Wellstart International. 1994. *Breastfeeding in Uganda: Beliefs and Practices*. Washington, D.C.: USAID.

Obermeyer, C. M., and S. Castle. 1997. Back to nature? Historical and cross-cultural perspectives on barriers to optimal breastfeeding. *Medical Anthropology* 17: 39–63.

O'Gara, Chloe, and Anna C. Martin. 1996. HIV and breast-feeding: Informed choice in the face of medical ambiguity. In *Women's Experiences with HIV/AIDS*, eds. Lynellyn D. Long and E. Maxine Ankrah. New York: Columbia University Press, pp. 220–235.

Panchula, Jeanette. 1998. WABA and pumps. Available from lactnet@library.ummed.edu; INTERNET, May 17.

Plank, S. J. and M. L. Milanesi. 1973. Infant feeding and mortality in rural Chile. *Bulletin of the World Health Organization* 48: 203–210.

Popkin, B. M. 1978. Economic determinants of breast feeding behavior: the case of rural households in Laguna, Philippines. In *Nutrition and Human Reproduction*, ed. W. H. Mosley. New York: Plenum, pp. 461–497.

Popkin, B. M., et al. 1990. Breast-feeding and diarrheal morbidity. *Pediatrics* 86: 874–882.

Raphael, Dana, and Flora Davis. 1985. *Only Mothers Know: Patterns of Infant Feeding in Traditional Cultures*. Westport, Conn.: Greenwood Press.

Ridler, Jean. 1996. Caution urged about assumptions related to breastfeeding women in Africa. *Journal of Human Lactation* 12: 11–12.

Ross, S. M., W. E. K. Loening and A. van Middelkoop. 1983. Breast-feeding: An evaluation of a health education programme. *South African Medical Journal* 64: 361–363.

Rubini, N. P., et al. 1994. Risks of bottle-feeding infants born to HIV-infected mothers from low-income families in Rio de Janeiro. Presented at the Tenth International Conference on AIDS, Yokohama, Japan, August 7–12. Abstract PCO158.

Ryder, R. W., et al. 1991. Evidence from Zaire that breast-feeding by HIV-1-seropositive mothers is not a major route for perinatal HIV-1 transmission but does decrease morbidity. *AIDS* 5: 709–714.

Saadeh, Randa J., Miriam H. Labbok, Kristin A. Cooney and Peggy Koniz-Booher,

eds. 1993. *Breast-feeding: The Technical Basis for Action*. Geneva, Switzerland: World Health Organization.

Saarinen, U. M., and M. Kajosaari. 1995. Breastfeeding as prophylaxis against atopic disease: Prospective follow-up study until 17 years old. *Lancet* 346: 1065–1069.

Savilahti, E., et al. 1987. Prolonged exclusive breastfeeding and heredity as determinants in infantile atopy. *Archives of Disease in Childhood* 62: 269–273.

Scariati, Paula D., Lawrence M. Grummer-Strawn and Sara Beck Fein. 1997. A longitudinal analysis of infant morbidity and the extent of breastfeeding in the United States. *Pediatrics* 99(6): e5.

Scarlett, D., et al. 1996. Breastfeeding prevalence among six-week-old infants at University Hospital of the West Indies. *West Indies Medical Journal* 45: 14–17.

Scott-Emuakpor, M. M., and U. A. Okafor. 1986. Comparative study of breastfed and bottlefed Nigerian infants. *East African Medical Journal* 63: 452–457.

Scrimshaw, Nevin S., C. E. Taylor and J. E. Gordon. 1968. *Interaction of Nutrition and Infection*. World Health Organization Monograph 57. Geneva.

Sepp, E., et al. 1997. Intestinal microflora of Estonian and Swedish infants. *Acta Paediatrica* 86: 956–961.

Shaffer, Nathan. 1998. Randomized placebo-controlled trial of short-course oral ZDV to reduce perinatal HIV transmission. Presented at the Twelfth World AIDS Conference, Geneva, Switzerland, June 28–July 3. Abstract 33163.

Stern, D. M. 1947. Prevention of epidemic neonatal diarrhoea. *Lancet*, January 11: 80–81.

Takala, A. K., et al. 1989. Risk factors of invasive Haemophilus influenzae type b disease among children in Finland. *Journal of Pediatrics* 115: 694–701.

Teka, T., A. S. G. Faruque and G. J. Fuchs. 1996. Risk factors for death in under-age-five children attending a diarrhoea treatment centre. *Acta Paediatrica* 85: 1070–1075.

Teele, David W., et al. 1989. Epidemiology of otitis media during the first seven years of life. *Journal of Infectious Diseases* 160: 83–95.

Tess, Beatriz H. 1997. Study of mother-to-infant transmission of HIV-1 in Brazil. Consultation on Infants and AIDS, Washington, D.C., July 17.

Tess, Beatriz H., et al. 1998. Breastfeeding, genetic, obstetric and other risk factors associated with mother-to-child transmission of HIV-1 in São Paulo State, Brazil. *AIDS* 12: 513–520.

U.S. Agency for International Development. 1990. *Breastfeeding: A Report on A.I.D. Programs*. Washington, D.C.: USAID.

UNICEF. 1998. Children: UNICEF backs breastfeeding over AIDS threat. *IPS Wire*, March 11.

UNICEF, UNAIDS, and the World Health Organization. 1998. *HIV and Infant Feeding: Guidelines for Decision-Makers*. Geneva, Switzerland: World Health Organization.

Urban, Mike. 1997. Attitudes and practices of infant feeding in HIV-1 infected women in Soweto. Presented at the Conference on Affordable Options for the Prevention of Mother-to-Child Transmission of HIV-1, Johannesburg, South Africa, November 19–20.

Van Esterik, Penny. 1988. The cultural context of infant feeding. In *Feeding Infants in Four Societies*, eds. Beverly Winikoff, Mary Ann Castle and Virginia Hight Laukaran. New York: Greenwood Press, pp. 187–201.

_____. 1989. *Beyond the Breast-Bottle Controversy*. New Brunswick, New Jersey: Rutgers University Press.

Victora, Cesar G., et al. 1987. Evidence for protection by breast-feeding against infant deaths from infectious diseases in Brazil. *Lancet* ii: 319–322.

Vis, Henri-L., Phillippe Hennart and Migabo Ruchababisha. 1981. Some issues in breast-feeding in deprived rural areas. *Assignment Children* 55/56: 183–200.

Wellstart International Expanded Promotion of Breastfeeding Program. 1994. *Final Report of Program in Rwanda, March 1992–April 1994*. Washington, D.C.: USAID.

Wold, A. E., and I. Adlerberth. 1998. Does breastfeeding affect the infant's immune responsiveness? (Invited commentary). *Acta Paediatrica* 87: 19–22.

Woods, Dave. 1997. A national dried milk formula. Presented at the Conference on Affordable Options for the Prevention of Mother-to-child Transmission of HIV-1, Johannesburg, South Africa, November 19–20.

World Health Assembly. 1994. *Infant and Young Child Nutrition*. Geneva: WHA 47.5.

_____. 1996. *Infant and Young Child Nutrition*. Geneva, Switzerland: WHA 49.15.

World Health Organization. 1991. Indicators for assessing breast-feeding practices. Report of an informal meeting, Geneva, Switzerland, June 11-12.

_____. 1996. *Breastfeeding Activities Progress Report*. Geneva, Switzerland: WHO.

Yoon, P. W., et al. 1996. Effect of not breastfeeding on the risk of diarrheal and respiratory mortality in children under 2 years of age in Metro Cebu, The Philippines. *American Journal of Epidemiology* 143: 1142–1148.

Young, H. B., et al. 1982. Milk and lactation: Some social and developmental correlates among 1,000 infants. *Pediatrics* 69: 169–175.

Zeitlin, M. F., M. Griffiths, R. K. Manoff and T. M. Cooke. 1984. Nutrition communication and behavioral change component. Volume IV. *Household Evaluation*. Indonesian Nutrition Development Program. Report by Manoff International, Inc., to Department of Health, Republic of Indonesia.

Zerfas, A. 1990. *Breastfeeding and Infant Feeding Graphs Based on Data from the Demographic Health Surveys*. Washington, D.C.: Academy for Educational Development.

Zohoori, Namvar, Barry M. Popkin and Maria E. Fernandez. 1993. Breast-feeding patterns in the Philippines: A prospective analysis. *Journal of Biosocial Science* 25: 127–138.

Zurayk, H. 1981. Breastfeeding and contraceptive patterns postpartum: A study in Lebanon. *Studies in Family Planning* 12: 237–247.

CHAPTER FIVE

---

# Don't We Want
# Women to Suckle So They
# Don't Get Pregnant Again?

While people in industrialized countries tend to think that women in resource-poor countries should breastfeed to keep their babies healthy, those who work in international programs are well aware that there is much more to breastfeeding than protection from diarrhea. Breastfeeding plays a role in controlling fertility, which may be one reason there has been reluctance to endorse alternative feeding methods, even for HIV-infected women. If HIV-infected women avoid breastfeeding and do not use contraceptives, they may soon become pregnant again and perhaps infect another baby.

Breastfeeding women don't menstruate or ovulate for varying lengths of time. Researchers reason, then, that breastfeeding keeps women infertile and spaces the intervals between births. Breastfeeding is still the major method of fertility control in countries where contraceptives are limited. The longer the interval between births, the greater the chances of survival for children in a resource-poor country (Hobcraft 1985). Professor Roger Short (1985) referred to breastfeeding as "Nature's Contraceptive" and noted that it has served us well for the last two million years. He also asserts that women in traditional societies seldom menstruated because they spent their reproductive lives either pregnant or lactating (producing breastmilk).

A woman who is not menstruating is called *amenorrheic*. If this is caused by lactation, it's called *lactational amenorrhea*. A woman who is not ovulating is said to be *anovulatory*. Although it is being anovulatory that prevents conception, most women do not know if they are anovulatory. So it is amenorrhea, or absence of menstruation, that is the practical guideline. Most, although not all, postpartum women menstruate before they ovulate.

## The Ovulation-Inhibiting Effect of Suckling

When a woman breastfeeds, the baby's sucking stimulation on her nipples does two main things. First, it "tells" her body to make milk (Tay 1996). Making enough milk is not primarily a matter of being motivated or well rested or drinking enough fluids, but is instead a matter of getting enough nipple stimulation and having milk removed at regular intervals. Bottle-feeding mothers dry up because they don't get nipple stimulation, and also because a local inhibiting factor in the residual milk "tells" their bodies not to make more milk (Daley 1996, Prentice 1989, Peaker 1995).

Secondly, in a separate pathway, nipple stimulation "tells" a woman's body not to release hormones that are needed for ovulation. The nipple stimulation sends signals to the woman's hypothalamus, which mediates the level and rhythm of hormones that control ovulation. It is the frequency and intensity of nipple stimulation that primarily controls a woman's return to fertility (Howie 1982b).

Babies who get semisolid foods may be not be hungry enough to suck intensely on their mothers' nipples. But semisolids do not seem as detrimental to continuing infertility as bottles (Huffman 1983). Breastfed babies who also get bottles tend to suck least often and least intensely. Sometimes mothers give so many bottles that their bodies get the message to stop making breastmilk.

Babies who suck on pacifiers (dummies) also tend to suck less avidly on their mothers' nipples. There is no hard evidence on this point, but it seems logical to advise noncontracepting mothers to direct their babies' sucking toward mothers' nipples, if they wish to remain infertile. One of the ten steps in UNICEF's current breastfeeding initiative specifically forbids pacifiers (dummies).

When breastfeeding women do become pregnant, they often stop breastfeeding. Under the influence of the hormones of pregnancy, a woman's milk supply dwindles and she often develops sore nipples. If her baby is fairly young when this happens, and the child is deprived of milk, it can be disastrous in settings where no good weaning foods are available. The woman who uses contraceptives, however, is generally able to breastfeed longer. Also, of course, contraceptives give women the desired control over their own fertility. Some women start using contraceptives after the time of natural infertility has ended, while others use them during natural infertility.

An effective way to enhance natural infertility is to promote cosleeping. When mothers and babies sleep together, babies usually nurse off and on all night, while both are asleep. In traditional societies, mothers and babies always slept together, as babies who did not cosleep risked death from predatory animals and hypothermia. Women who now practice cosleeping tend to remain infertile for a considerable period of time, even if their babies receive lots of other foods during the day. Women who breastfeed off and on, both all day and all night, tend to have the most prolonged infertility.

## The Extreme in Breastfeeding Frequency

In societies where women breastfeed very frequently, they usually have children at intervals of two years or longer. The 1980 report from Konner and Worthman reveals that the !Kung, hunter-gatherers in Botswana and Namibia, use no contraceptives during frequent sexual relations and have a birth interval of 4.1 years. !Kung mothers breastfeed their babies so frequently that they start a new breastfeeding session every 13 minutes, on average. Most breastfeeding sessions are extremely brief, only two to three minutes in duration. So every 13 minutes, a !Kung woman puts her child to breast again, for another two–three minute breastfeeding session. This pattern is not limited to young babies, but continues for children up to the age of 139 weeks. The longest interval between feeding, as observed by Harvard University anthropologists, was 55 minutes. All mothers reported that their children nursed during the night without waking them.

Although this pattern of very short, very frequent nursing strikes many people in industrialized countries as strange, it is probably the norm for earlier societies. The fact that human milk is extremely dilute may also explain why very frequent nursing is normal. By contrast, mammals with very concentrated milk go much longer between feeding sessions. The tree shrew, which has very concentrated milk, nurses her young only once every 48 hours (Ben Shaul 1962).

Most babies who are fed only human milk appear inclined to suckle frequently, whereas babies who get other foods can go longer between feedings, allowing mothers to do other things and explaining why many overworked women give their babies other foods. But women who do not breastfeed exclusively are less likely to receive the nipple stimulation they need to stay infertile. Women do not have to restrict their intervals between breastfeeding sessions to 13 minutes, however, in order to remain infertile, at least not in the early months. Most women will remain amenorrheic in the first six months with a nursing frequency of 10 daily episodes, especially if they cosleep (Howie 1982c).

## Prevention of Millions of Births

According to data collected between 1974 and 1984, the amount of fertility inhibited by breastfeeding varied greatly according to the style of breastfeeding (Thapa 1988). In sub–Saharan Africa, breastfeeding reduced fertility by four births per woman. If breastfeeding in the region had then declined by only 25 percent, contraceptive use would have had to increase by nearly 150 percent to keep fertility rates constant. By contrast, women in many Asian and Latin American countries breastfed less intensely and lactational anovulation prevented a smaller proportion of births. If breastfeeding in Asia had declined by 25 percent, it would have taken only a 23 percent increase in use of contraceptives to compensate. If breastfeeding in Latin America had declined by 25 percent, it would have taken only a 5 percent increase in use of contraceptives.

According to a 1989 WHO report, breastfeeding-related infertility is so significant that it would require a fivefold increase in contraceptives just to maintain the current fertility rates if women in resource-poor countries breastfed as little as women in industrialized countries do (WHO 1989). Short (1991) reported that breastfeeding in Africa has been preventing more births than all other forms of contraception combined. The average African woman gives birth to six children, with five more prevented by breastfeeding.

Since data were collected between 1974 and 1984, some women have moved away from the pattern of intense suckling. Daily episodes of suckling declined when women began to work away from their babies in distant fields or at other jobs. As women became more urbanized, had more education and used more contraceptives, these factors also contributed to less breastfeeding (Grummer-Strawn 1996). Use of contraceptives was also noted to have increased in rural Zimbabwe, as 37 percent of married women were using them (Gregson 1998). But if women in Africa or India, for example, gave up breastfeeding (because of HIV), many would be likely to become pregnant again much sooner. Many more contraceptives would need to be made available and would need to be used. The prospect of losing breastfeeding-related infertility is daunting.

According to UNICEF, however, the funding needed to expand family planning services "stands in almost absurd contrast to the smallness of the resources required." In fact, UNICEF's James Grant noted in 1994 noted that the current family planning services account for less than half of 1 percent of government spending in the developing world, and less than 1.5 percent of all aid from governments in the industrialized world.

## Lactational Amenorrhea and Malnutrition

In general, women under 30 years of age and well-nourished women resume fertility cycles earlier. When a mother is so severely malnourished that her breastmilk supply starts to decline, her baby will suck more frequently in an attempt to make up the deficit. This extra nipple stimulation prolongs the duration of infertility (Short 1993). Huffman (1983) described lactational amenorrhea among women in Bangladesh, noting that thin, poorly nourished mothers averaged 20.2 months of lactational amenorrhea, compared to 15.5 months for better-nourished women. Nutritional status, however, is less significant than the effect of nipple stimulation in determining the duration of her amenorrhea.

The Bangladeshi mothers tended to resume menstruation and ovulation during the harvest season, when their children were toddlers. Thus subsequent births tended to be clustered together, nine months after harvest. There are several possible reasons why the women ovulated during harvest season. First, they were likely to be getting less nipple stimulation during the day because they were too busy harvesting to sit and nurse their toddlers. Decreased nipple stimulation is often followed by resumed ovulation. Secondly, the malnourished Bangladeshi women, who were nursing toddlers, were likely to have been producing fairly little milk. After they were better nourished with foods available at harvest, they may have made more milk, so their children needed to suck less intensely to get enough milk. Thirdly, perhaps because they finally got enough to eat, the mothers may have built up their body fat enough to ovulate. The effect of malnutrition on menstruation was established during the famines associated with the two World Wars. People talked about *l'aménorrhée de famine* and also about *Kriegs-ammenorrheën*, or "war amenorrhea" (Hennart and Vis 1980). Anorexic girls who lose their body fat also become amenorrheic.

But the Bangladeshi women still averaged a year and a half of lactational amenorrhea, which kept their children from being displaced too soon by a younger sibling. The West African name *kwashiorkor* literally means the deprivation of a child who is no longer breastfed because his mother has become pregnant again (Williams 1938). Children in resource-poor countries who are displaced early by a new sibling have significantly higher mortality rates than children whose mothers have longer birth intervals. (Hobcraft 1985).

Lactational amenorrhea also helps women to avoid anemia by allowing their bodies to replenish iron stores. It is women who spend much of their reproductive years in an anovulatory state (because of repeated pregnancies and lactations) who truly have low rates of ovarian cancer and postmenopausal breast cancer.

## Different Styles of Breastfeeding

A study of infant feeding in four societies (Winikoff 1988) explained very well how different breastfeeding styles affect fertility. Two of the sites

(Bangkok, Thailand, and Nairobi, Kenya) now have high rates of HIV sero-prevalence and are therefore particularly relevant to projections about the likely effects on fertility if HIV-infected women avoid breastfeeding.

In Bangkok, 90 percent of the mothers initiated breastfeeding, but many stopped early on. In the first 29 days after delivery, only 76 percent of the mothers were breastfeeding at all. From four months on, only 40–45 percent still breastfed. Exclusive breastfeeding was rare, and, as a result, the median duration of amenorrhea was only 2.88 months. This is not much longer than the eight weeks of lactational amenorrhea that Scottish bottle-feeders experienced (Howie 1982a). Since contraceptives were fairly accessible, however, the loss of lactational amenorrhea had no discernible effect on population growth in Thailand. Thailand, in fact, is expected to see its population decrease because of AIDS.

At the Nairobi site, researchers found that all mothers breastfed, although 85 percent supplemented by three months postpartum. The researchers noted that, although mothers in *rural* Kenya nursed frequently day and night, *urban* mothers nursed much less frequently. They felt that this almost certainly contributed to a shorter-than-expected length of amenorrhea (only 6–9 months). From birth to four months, 91 percent of the mothers who were solely breastfeeding were amenorrheic. Of mothers who fed other milks and solids in addition to breastmilk, 68 percent were amenorrheic. Of those who did not breastfeed at all, 60 percent still did not menstruate. From 5 to 9 months, 64 percent of full breastfeeders, 49 percent of the mixed-feeders, and only 24 percent of the nonbreastfeeders were amenorrheic.

Breastfeeding has been the traditional restraint on population growth in countries such as Kenya. But because breastfeeding duration and postpartum sexual abstinence have both declined and contraceptives are not widely used, Kenya now has one of the highest growth rates in the world (Saadeh and Benbouzid 1997). They noted also that in some countries such as Mexico, Columbia and Zaire, amenorrhea lasts only three or four months. In India and Haiti the duration is twelve months.

## High Partial Breastfeeding — It's Not Just for Babies

A report from rural Zaire (Vis 1981) showed how beneficial semitraditional breastfeeding is for fertility control, even though it may not be particularly effective at keeping babies healthy. The report described a pattern of feeding that seems to best fit the definition of high partial breastfeeding. That is, although the babies were only *partially* breastfed, they received *high* amounts of breastmilk. According to the report, malnutrition in Zaire was widespread, especially among children and pregnant and breastfeeding women. As with many cultures with too little food, men were served first, then children, and women last. When pregnant, these women in rural Zaire gained on average only 2–3 kilograms (4.4–6.6 pounds). They ranged in age from 16 to 48 years, and had between 1 and 14 children, with an average of 5.

The women nursed 9–17 times per day at one month postpartum, 6-27 times each day at 12 months and 6–25 times per day at 24 months. Given the very large number of breastfeeds and the malnutrition, it is not surprising that most women remained amenorrheic for a long time. At one year after childbirth, only 19 percent of the women were menstruating regularly. At 18 months after childbirth, only 25 percent of the women were menstruating regularly. By two years after birth, 60 percent of the children were still nursing, and 80 percent of the mothers were menstruating. The birth intervals were long, with about 33–39 months between births.

By the second or third week mothers had begun feeding bananas, boiled sorghum or manioc paste, prechewing and then hand-feeding them to their babies. When asked why they introduced the foods, the women often replied, "The child is crying from hunger and there is not enough milk." Some women also worked in fields far from home and left their babies all day in the care of a grandmother or a sister, who fed the same foods. Following the introduction of solids, the first signs of gastroenteritis and parasitic infections appeared. Some of the babies were said to suffer "disastrous effects." Some died. If asked why they left their babies all day, the women pointed to the great distances from their homes to the fields. High partial breastfeeding, in this case, then, served better the mothers' interests than the babies', proving more effective at controlling fertility than at keeping children well.

## Women's Changing Lives

The women in rural Zaire in the late 1970s were not unusual in that they were prevented by work from breastfeeding as frequently as their mothers and grandmothers had. More women in recent generations have been working in shops and factories, and on the larger agricultural tracts that produce crops for export. Women are also drawn to aspects of Western culture, although only people with money can afford to buy Western clothing, Coca-Cola, infant formula, or commercial baby cereals.

While many women still cosleep with their babies, however, an increasing number of them are either unable or unwilling to adopt the intense style of breastfeeding necessary for natural infertility. While lactational amenorrhea continues to postpone pregnancy on a population basis, it is not completely reliable on an individual basis. People in many societies have noted that some women become pregnant again even while they are fully breastfeeding young babies. Most people interviewed in Uganda, in fact, thought that breastfeeding was unrelated to birth intervals. According to USAID, in such regions nursing "does not help even those who breastfeed 10 times a day" (Nutrition Division, Wellstart 1994). Some Westerners have also questioned whether it is sound public health policy to recommend lactational amenorrhea as a contraceptive (Trussell 1991, UNFPA 1990).

Women who breastfeed briefly are unlikely to achieve much or any protection from pregnancy because they would have been infertile in the early weeks anyway. A carefully conducted study in Scotland showed that bottle-feeding mothers began to menstruate at approximately 8 weeks after delivery and began to ovulate at approximately 10.8 weeks (Howie 1982a).

In the late 1990s some researchers began to suggest that HIV-infected women in very poor areas breastfeed for only a few months, hoping that this will preserve some of the benefits of breastfeeding and still reduce the risk of HIV transmission. But three months of breastfeeding would not lengthen the duration of infertility much beyond total bottle-feeding.

## Are Sucking Babies Useful?

In her book, *The Politics of Breastfeeding*, Gabrielle Palmer asks, "Are dead babies useful?" as she examines the attitude of people who see the deaths of Third World babies as a natural or even useful part of population control. By the same token, one can ask: Are sucking babies useful? In delaying their mothers' return to ovulation, sucking babies are very useful, and HIV-infected babies may be especially useful. When children do not feel well, they tend to suck more (Black 1982, Delgado 1982, Hoyle 1980). Frequent sucking at the breast may be due to a desire for comfort or a diarrhea-driven thirst (Huffman 1983). When mothers perceive that their children are sickly, they tend to continue breastfeeding longer, even at the expense of their own comfort (Marquis and Rasmussen 1996). So HIV-infected mothers who are breastfeeding sick HIV-infected children are likely to average many months of natural infertility.

## Postpartum Abstinence

People long ago adapted their behaviors to the biology of pregnancy and breastfeeding. People in earlier civilizations knew that if a breastfeeding mother became pregnant, her milk supply dwindled. If this happened too soon after delivery, and if the family lived in a society with no good alternatives to breastfeeding, the baby stood a substantial risk of dying. This led people to declare breastfeeding mothers off limits to sexual intercourse. This postpartum abstinence was especially important in cultures where breastfeeding was less intense. Women such as the !Kung, who breastfeed every 13 minutes, do not need taboos on intercourse. But there are many cultures in which women breastfeed more to "feed" their babies or put them to sleep than to comfort them.

Postpartum taboos on intercourse have always been the backup method. In some cultures taboos on intercourse lasted for as long as a child nursed; this was often three years or even longer. In other cultures, taboos governed just the early months of breastfeeding. In Moslem tradition, couples could resume intercourse 40 days after childbirth. Men who felt deprived because their wives were off limits, perhaps for two years, coped by taking on additional wives. Polygamy became fairly common.

Dr. Sandra Gray (1995) reported an interesting example of polygamy and breastfeeding working together. She described a group of nomadic pastoralists who tended animals in rural Kenya. They lived by frequently moving their camels, cattle, sheep, goats and donkeys in search of water and vegetation. Since successful herders needed multiple wives and children to tend the animals, polygamy was common. As might be expected, young children depended on breastfeeding. When the women grew weary of nursing their toddlers, they would decide to wean. Weaning , however, is not so easy for women who sleep with their children. Gray noted that a woman might wean by sending her child to sleep with a co-wife. The woman who was relieved of breastfeeding would then take on the task of having sex with the shared husband.

Polygamy protected women from premature pregnancies and, because women often stop breastfeeding when they know they are pregnant, spared young children from losing their mothers' milk. But not everyone saw the value of polygamy. Christian missionaries disapproved of the practice and told women to stop abstaining postpartum. This was supposed to encourage men to have only one sexual partner (their wives), and to protect the men's mortal souls. While abandonment of postpartum abstinence was good for Church teaching, it was not so good for either the women who became pregnant sooner or the babies, who often lost their mothers' milk before they were ready. From the fifteenth to the eighteenth century in Europe, Church authorities who were concerned with the husbands' mortal souls had recommended that babies be wet nursed so that wives could resume sexual relations (Obermeyer 1997). No mention was made of the souls of the of the wet nurses' husbands.

AIDS is now leading some people to call again for an end to polygamy. Women's rights activists of Zambia have recommended the motto "one man one woman" as a way of encouraging the development of a monogamous society (Namanza 1997). Dr. Olive Ssentumbwe Mugisha, head of Uganda's Women's Doctors Association, called for a bill that would limit the maximum number of wives to two (Polygamy 1998).

AIDS is also changing some taboos on intercourse. Researchers from Wellstart (Nutrition Division 1994) noted that the Itesots of Uganda used to believe that breastfeeding women should abstain from sexual contact for about two years and that men should be allowed to sleep with other women. But AIDS changed public opinion: "With the advent of the AIDS epidemic, the women said, more couples are breaking the taboo so that the man will not seek an outside partner, causing some women to get pregnant again when their babies were still young." It should be noted, however, that if mothers become pregnant while their infants still suckle, their breastfeeding practices may not be compatible with lactational amenorrhea.

In Zimbabwe, as well, there has been a call for the end of postpartum abstinence. Thomasmoore Chaita, the health ministry's director of child nutrition service, noted that abstinence during pregnancy and in the first few months of breastfeeding is no longer advisable because "partners are likely to look for sexual satisfaction from other women who may be infected with HIV" (Machekanyange 1997). Women in rural Zimbabwe now also resume sex early after childbirth to avoid having their mates take other partners (Gregson 1998). Other women are choosing to breastfeed less in order to reduce postpartum abstinence and encourage their husbands to remain faithful (Greiner 1994).

## LAM

The natural ovulation-inhibiting effect of breastfeeding was "codified" as LAM (the Lactational Amenorrhea Method), an official method of family planning. At the 1988 Bellagio (Italy) Consensus Conference, scientists agreed that amenorrheic women who were fully or almost fully breastfeeding in the first six months and who were amenorrheic were likely to experience a risk of pregnancy of only two percent (Kennedy 1989). Dr. Miriam Labbok and colleagues codified LAM at Georgetown University in 1989. Experts concluded in 1995 that the Bellagio consensus had been confirmed by these additional studies (Kennedy 1996).

LAM has three specific conditions (amenorrhea, in the first six months, with frequent suckling) and has been made easy for health workers to use with mothers. The health worker asks three questions:

(1) Have your menses returned? (Bleeding in the first 56 days or spotting does not count.)
(2) Are you supplementing breastfeeding or allowing long periods of time without breastfeeding, day or night? (Intervals between feeds should not exceed four hours in the daytime or six hours at night. Ideally, breastfeeding should be exclusive but small amounts of supplements do not interfere as long as the baby is sucking frequently.)
(3) Is your baby older than six months? (Frequent breastfeeding by older babies can also delay ovulation, but is only recently becoming part of LAM.)

When a mother answers yes to any of the three questions, she is to be advised to begin using another family planning method. With LAM, women need to meet all three criteria in order to consider themselves infertile. Additionally, women who begin to give more than token amounts of food or liquids other than breastmilk should begin to use a contraceptive if they wish to avoid pregnancy. LAM necessitates breastfeeding during the night and close proximity of mother and child day and night (Labbok 1997). Some women, however, have early return to menses despite such frequent nursing.

## USAID's Breastfeeding/LAM Programs

Although UNICEF and the World Health Organization are the most well known players in international breastfeeding circles, there are other major organizations and funders. One is USAID, the United States Agency for International Development. Funded by the Office of Population, USAID spends millions of dollars on breastfeeding programs and research that emphasize family planning (USAID 1990). The agency's breastfeeding programs in Africa, Latin America and Asia utilized "breastfeeding promotion in the context of fertility services" (Huffman and Labbok 1994).

Population monitoring is a major activity of USAID, with its health and education focuses serving primarily its population control objectives (Hartman 1995:114). The agency's multicenter study of LAM gathered data prospectively in 11 sites in 1994-1995, including Egypt, Indonesia, Mexico, Nigeria (Jos), Nigeria (Sagamu), Philippines, Germany, Italy, Sweden, United Kingdom, and the United States (Labbok 1997).

LAM is especially welcome where contraceptives are little used for reasons ranging from lack of funding to Catholic Church policies. Those who feel the need to have many children, in hopes that a few will survive to adulthood, do not generally use contraceptives but may be convinced to breastfeed intensely for lengthening birth intervals.

Silvia Catalán, professor of pediatrics at Catholic University in Chile, reported the success of a program in which she and colleagues worked with women living in an area where the influence of the Catholic Church over government policies had limited the availability of contraceptives. By establishing a program to show women how to breastfeed in such a way as to remain infertile, Catalán and colleagues (1996) were able to increase the incidence of exclusive breastfeeding to an incredible 66 percent. Women seemed more willing to breastfeed intensely when they also felt that there was something — such as prolonged infertility — in it for them. Earlier programs in Chile (Diaz 1982, Valdez 1990) had also supported breastfeeding "in the context of fertility services"(Saadeh 1993:37). A project in Ecuador offered breastfeeding services in family-planning clinics and found that women were willing to pay for breastfeeding as "a means of child spacing" (Sevilla 1991). Women in Yemen also indicated that the reason they breastfed longer was to achieve greater birth spacing (Greiner 1983).

The efforts involved in increasing the duration and intensity of breastfeeding have often been extensive. In Chile, the Ministry of Health and others trained health teams and mothers in the management of breastfeeding. They established breastfeeding clinics in primary health care centers, initiated UNICEF's Baby Friendly Hospital Initiative, and modernized study programs for health care workers. They instituted some provisions of the WHO Code to limit formula advertising (Castillo 1996). But it was the women unable to get contraceptives who were most likely to breastfeed intensely.

## HIV/AIDS and Issues of Fertility

A call has been made for programs to supply contraceptives for non-breastfeeding women. But concern has been raised, based on a study of monkeys (Marx 1996) and some small studies of women, that progesterone-based contraceptives (the pill and Depo-Provera) may increase the likelihood of a woman's becoming HIV-infected. Policymakers will wait until more research is available before considering changes in recommendations, but if progesterone contraceptives become less recommended, then the loss of lactational amenorrhea would be doubly unwelcome.

While the number of tested, HIV-positive women is as yet too tiny to have an impact on fertility rates, abandonment of breastfeeding by untested mothers might significantly affect them. Professor John Cleland (1996) of the Centre for Population Studies noted that the world population is increasing by 90 million per year and that the traditional scourges of mankind (famine, warfare and pestilence) are unlikely to slow the growth. Birth rates, then, have a greater effect on the population than death rates. High birth rates used to be balanced with high mortality rates. Now, however, mortality rates have decreased with the spread of programs for mass immunizations and oral rehydration (which helps prevent death from dehydration). Cleland estimated that a group would have to have a seroprevalence of 40–50 percent to cancel out a population growth of 3 percent per year.

Although the overall impact of AIDS on slowing world population growth is likely to be minor, recent research suggests that AIDS will have a greater impact on the populations of certain high-risk areas than was originally thought. For Uganda, the population was impacted "much earlier than previously imagined" (Low-Beer 1997). Prevalence in Uganda has declined because of successful educational strategies, but also because so many people have died or moved away (Wawer 1997). In one area, approximately 9 percent of HIV-infected women of childbearing age have died each year (Serwadda 1996).

HIV-positive women in Kenya (Nyange 1992), Zaire (Ryder 1991), and Uganda (Widy-Wirski 1988) were reported to be less fertile. Dr. Ronald Gray (1997, 1998) reported that Ugandan women who were HIV-positive were significantly less likely to be fertile, especially if their HIV disease was symptomatic. In fact, women who were HIV-positive and asymptomatic stood only a 67 percent chance of becoming pregnant, while symptomatic women had only a 36 percent chance. The rate of pregnancy loss was significantly greater for HIV-positive women, as 18.5 percent of them lost a pregnancy, compared to 12.2 percent of HIV-negative women. Whether or not women were aware of their HIV status had no effect. The pregnancy rate among HIV-1-positive women was 14.2 percent, compared to 21.4 percent among HIV-1-negative women (Gray 1998).

This study suggests also that seroprevalence is higher than has been believed. Researchers often base estimates of seroprevalence in resource-poor countries on blood tests of pregnant women. If HIV-positive women are relatively infertile, then there are likely more HIV-positive women who are not pregnant. Figures based on pregnant women are likely to seriously underestimate the prevalence in Uganda (Wawer 1997) and in Tanzania (Kigadve 1993).

## Women's Reactions to High HIV Prevalence

The women who live in Uganda and Tanzania and other severely affected countries do not need to read seroprevalence figures to know that AIDS is increasing mortality rates. In Uganda, for example, AIDS caused 7 out of every 10 deaths for men 25–44 years old and for women aged 20–44 (UNAIDS 1997). The experience of watching great numbers of deaths does not lead people to want fewer babies. On the contrary, anthropologists tell us that after wars there is "an almost atavistic urge to reproduce"— evidenced in the United States by the baby boom following World War I — as people naturally follow the patterns of ancestors (Tobias 1997:67).

Women who see the AIDS-associated increases in deaths, then, may have more, not fewer, births (Carovano 1991). One HIV-infected woman said, "I don't mind dying, but to die without a child means that I will have perished without a trace" (Barnett 1990). In some cultures, a person who dies without leaving successors is barred from being accepted as an ancestral spirit. In rural Zimbabwe, the epidemic was described as being in fairly early stages, compared to urban areas, and observers have not yet seen any strong upward pressure on fertility due to conscious replacement efforts (Gregson 1998).

Carovano also pointed out that in many societies, it is motherhood that brings validation and security to women's lives. She quoted a young woman in Uganda, who when asked why she was not protecting herself from HIV replied, "Babies and condoms don't go together, nonpenetrative sex is no sex at all for a man, and it is a woman's responsibility to bear a child."

Some people in resource-poor countries such as Uganda have seen family-planning methods as a "western plot" to control Third World population (Lyons 1997:142). In South Africa, some people associate family planning messages with "genocidal conspiracy allegations" (Van der Vliet 1994). People who see condom promotion efforts as another imperialist racist attempt at population control aren't likely to use condoms.

Carovano (1991) noted another problem: "To provide women exclusively with HIV prevention methods that contradict most societies' fertility norms is to provide many women with no options at all." To date, all methods that protect against HIV infection also prevent pregnancy. Female-controlled HIV prevention products such as vaginal microbicides are still under development. AIDS programs are now distributing female condoms by the millions, and there is hope that they will be more widely accepted than traditional male condoms. But unlike microbicides, female condoms are quite visible. It has been suggested that female condoms be distributed for women to use while breastfeeding, given that the risk of infecting a breastfeeding baby is great following sero-conversion. One would hope that nonbreastfeeding mothers and women who are not pregnant would be considered worthy of protection for their own sake.

Keeping mothers from becoming HIV-infected while breastfeeding and keeping new mothers from becoming pregnant again are two major challenges. Programs that provide formula for babies of HIV-infected women would be wise to help mothers prevent unwanted pregnancies. As UNICEF's James Grant has noted, the amount of funding needed to supply contraceptives is comparatively small.

While lactational amenorrhea has served humankind well for millions of years and will continue to do so for many women, the infant feeding policy for HIV-infected women is supposed to be informed choice. It seems unlikely that infected (or worried) women will choose to feed their babies potentially infectious breastmilk just to keep themselves temporarily infertile. Offering them counseling and contraceptives would be more appropriate.

# References

Barnett, T., et al. 1990. Community coping mechanisms in the face of exceptional demographic change. Final report to the Overseas Development Administration.

Ben Shaul, D. M. 1962. The composition of the milk of wild animals. *International Zoology Yearbook* 4: 333–342.

Black, R. E., K. Brown, S. Becker and M. Yunus. 1982. Longitudinal studies of infectious diseases and physical growth of children in rural Bangladesh: Patterns of morbidity. *American Journal of Epidemiology* 115: 305–314.

Bonte, M., et al. 1974. Influence of the socio-economic level on the conception rate during lactation. *International Journal of Fertility* 19: 97–102.

Carovano, Kathryn. 1991. More than mothers and whores: Redefining the AIDS prevention needs of women. *International Journal of Health Sciences* 21: 131–142.

Castillo, Cecilia, Eduardo Atalah, José Riumalló and René Castro. 1996. Breastfeeding and the nutritional status of nursing children in Chile. *Bulletin of PAHO* 30: 125–133.

Catalán, Silvia. 1996. Pre-service training. Presented at the Colloquium on Training in Breastfeeding Programmes, Bangkok, Thailand, November 24–30.

Cleland, John. 1996. Population growth in the 21st century cause for crisis or celebration? *Tropical Medicine and International Health* 1: 15–26.

Daley, Steven J., Jacqueline C. Kent, Robyn A. Owens and Peter E. Hartman. 1996. Frequency and degree of milk removal and the short-term control of human milk synthesis. *Experimental Physiology* 81: 861–875.

Delgado, H., R. Martorell and R. E. Klein. 1982. Nutrition, lactation and birth interval components in rural Guatemala. *American Journal of Clinical Nutrition* 35: 1468–1476.

Diaz, S., et al. 1982. Fertility regulation in nursing women. *Journal of Biosocial Science* 14: 329.

Grant, James P. 1994. *The State of the World's Children.* New York: UNICEF.

Gray, Ronald H. 1997. Impact of HIV infection on fertility. Presented at the Conference on Global Strategies for the Prevention of HIV Transmission from Mothers to Infants, Washington, D.C., September 3–6.

Gray, R. H., et al. 1998. Population-based study of fertility in women with HIV-1 in Uganda. *Lancet* 351: 98–103.

Gray, Sandra. 1995. Correlates of breastfeeding frequency among Nomadic pastoralists of Turkana, Kenya: A retrospective study. *American Journal of Physical Anthropology* 98: 239–255.

Gregson, Simon, Tom Zhuwau, Roy M. Anderson and Stephen K. Chandiwana. 1998. Is there evidence for behavior change in response to AIDS in rural Zimbabwe? *Social Science and Medicine* 46: 321–330.

Greiner, Ted. 1994. Sustained breastfeeding, complementation and care. Revised and condensed version of a "Focus Paper" for the Cornell UNICEF Expert Working Group Colloquium on Care and Nutrition for the Young Child, Aurora, New York, October 12–15.

Grummer-Strawn, Lawrence M. 1996. The effect of changes in population characteristics on breastfeeding trends in fifteen resource-poor countries. *International Journal of Epidemiology* 25: 94–102.

Hartman, Betsy. 1995. *Reproductive Rights and Wrongs: The Global Politics of Population Control.* Boston: South End Press.

Hennart, P., and H. L. Vis. 1980. Breast-feeding and postpartum amenorrhea in central Africa. I. Milk production in rural areas. *Journal of Tropical Pediatrics* 26: 171–183.

Hobcraft, J. N., J. W. McDonald and S. O. Rutstein. 1985. Demographic determinants of infant and early child mortality: A comparative analysis. *Population Studies* 39: 363–385.

Howie, P. W., et al. 1982a. Fertility after childbirth: Infant feeding patterns, basal PRL levels and post-partum ovulation. *Clinical Endocrinology* 17: 315–322.

_____. 1982b. Fertility after childbirth: Post-partum ovulation and menstruation in bottle and breast feeding mothers. *Clinical Endocrinology* 17: 323–332.

Howie, P. W., and A. S. McNeilly. 1982c. Effect of breast feeding patterns on human birth intervals. *Journal of Reproduction and Fertility* 65: 545–557.

Hoyle, Bruce, M. Yunus and Lincoln C. Chen. 1980. Breast-feeding and food intake among children with acute diarrheal disease. *American Journal of Clinical Nutrition* 33: 2365–2371.

Huffman, Sandra L. 1983. Maternal and child nutritional status: Its association with the risk of pregnancy. *Social Science and Medicine* 17: 1529–1540.

Huffman, S. L., and M. H. Labbok. 1994. Breastfeeding in family planning programs: A help or a hindrance? *International Journal of Gynaecology and Obstetrics* 47 (Supplement) S23–31.

Kennedy, K. I., R. Rivera and A. McNeilly. 1989. Consensus statement on the use of breastfeeding as a family planning method. *Contraception* 39: 477–496.

Kennedy, K. I., M. H. Labbok and P. F. A. Van Look. 1996. Consensus statement lactational amenorrhea method for family planning. *International Journal of Obstetrics and Gynecology* 54: 55–57.

Kigadve, R. M., et. al. 1993. Sentinel surveillance for HIV-1 among pregnant women in a resource-poor country: 3 years' experience and comparison with a population seropositivity. *AIDS* 7: 849–855.

Konner, Melvin, and Carol Worthman. 1980. Nursing frequency, gonadal function, and birth spacing among !Kung hunter-gatherers. *Science* 207: 788–791.

Labbok, Miriam H., et al. 1997. Multicenter study of the lactational amenorrhea method (LAM): I. Efficiency, duration and implications for clinical application. *Contraception* 55: 327–336.

Low-Beer, D., et al. 1997. Empirical evidence for the severe but localized impact of AIDS on population structure. *Nature Medicine* 3: 553–557.

Lyons, Maryinez. 1997. The point of view: Perspectives on AIDS in Uganda. In *AIDS in Africa and the Caribbean*, eds. George C. Bond, John Kreniske, Ida Susser and Joan Vincent. Boulder, Colorado: Westview Press, pp. 131–146.

Machekanyange, Zorodzai. 1997. Zimbabwe: Is breast milk still best? *Africa Information Afrique*. Harare, Zimbabwe, September 8.

Marquis, Grace S., and Kathleen M. Rasmussen. 1996. Extended breastfeeding and malnutrition: An example of reverse causality. In *Exclusive Breastfeeding Promotion: A Summary from EPB's Applied Research Program (1992–1996)*. USAID.

Marquis, Grace S., et al. 1998. Association of breastfeeding and stunting to Peruvian toddlers: An example of reverse causality. *International Journal of Epidemiology* 26: 349–356.

Marx, Preston A., et al. 1996. Progesterone implants enhance SIV vaginal transmission and early viral load. *Nature Medicine* 2: 1084–1089.

Namanza, Dickson. 1997. Zambian women oppose polygamy. Xinhua New Agency, April 26.

Nutrition Division of the Uganda Ministry of Health, Child Health and Development Center of Makerere University and Wellstart International. 1994. *Breastfeeding in Uganda: Beliefs and Practices.* Washington, D.C.: USAID.

Nyange, P. M., P. Datta. J. Embree and J. O. Ndinya-Achola. 1992. Morbidity and mortality in HIV infected African women. Presented at the Eighth International Conference on AIDS, Amsterdam, Netherlands, July 19–24. Abstract POC 4373.

Obermeyer, C. M., and S. Castle. 1997. Back to nature? Historical and cross-cultural perspectives on barriers to optimal breastfeeding. *Medical Anthropology* 17: 39–63.

Palmer, Gabrielle. 1993. *The Politics of Breastfeeding.* London: Pandora Press.

Peaker, Malcolm. 1995. Autocrine control of milk secretion: Development of the concept. In *Intercellular Signaling in the Mammary Gland,* eds. C. J. Wilde, et al. New York: Pleneum Press, pp. 193–202.

Polygamy Contributes to AIDS Deaths in Uganda. 1998. *Africa News Service,* April 6.

Prentice, Ann, Caroline V. P. Addey and Colin J. Wilde. 1989. Evidence for local feedback control of human milk secretion. *Biochemical Society Transactions* 17: 122.

Ryder, R. W., et al. 1991. Fertility rates in 238 HIV-1 seropositive women in Zaire followed for 3 years postpartum. *AIDS* 5: 1521–1527.

Saadeh, R., and D. Benbouzid. 1990. Breast-feeding and child-spacing: Importance of information collection for public health policy. *Bulletin of the World Health Organization* 68: 623–631.

Saadeh, Randa J., Miriam H. Labbok, Kristin A. Cooney and Peggy Koniz-Booher, eds. 1993. *Breastfeeding: The Technical Basis for Action.* Geneva, Switzerland: World Health Organization.

Serwadda, David, et al. 1996. HIV-1 incidence and prevalence among pregnant women in a population-based rural cohort, Rakai District, Uganda. Eleventh International Conference on AIDS, Vancouver, Canada, July 7–12. Abstract Th.C.344.

Sevilla, F. 1991. CEMOPLAF *Final Report on the Introduction of* LAM *into a Multi-Method Family Planning Delivery System.* Washington, D.C.: Georgetown University.

Short, Roger. 1985. Nature's contraceptive. *Journal of Biosocial Science* 9: 1–3.

_____. 1991. Report at a UN Administrative Committee on Coordination Subcommittee on Nutrition. Reported in *New & Noteworthy* (no. 15), ed. Alan Berg, November 13.

_____. 1993. Lactational infertility in family planning. *Annals of Medicine* 25: 175–180.

Tay, C. C. K., A. F. Glasier and A. S. McNeilly. 1996. Twenty-four hour patterns of prolactin secretion during lactation and the relationship to suckling and the resumption of fertility in breast-feeding women. *Human Reproduction* 11: 950–955.

Thapa, Shyam, Roger V. Short and Malcolm Potts. 1988. Breast feeding, birth spacing and their effects on child survival. *Nature* 335: 679–682.

Tobias, Sheila. 1997. *Faces of Feminism*. Boulder, Colorado: Westview Press.

Trussell, J., and G. Santow. 1991. Is the Bellagio consensus statement on the use of contraception sound public-health policy? *Health Transition Review* 1: 105–114.

U.S. Agency for International Development. 1990. *Breastfeeding: A Report on A.I.D. Programs*. Washington, D.C.: USAID.

_____. *About USAID*. Available at http://www.info.usaid.gov/about; INTERNET.

UNAIDS. 1997. *Report on the Global HIV/AIDS Epidemic*. Geneva, Switzerland: UNAIDS.

United Nations Fund for Population Activities. 1990. Pledging support, Sadik warns of breastfeeding trap. *Population* 16(9): 1.

Valdez, V., and A. Perez. 1990. *Lactancia Materna*. Washington, D.C.: The Institute for Reproductive Health, Georgetown University.

Van der Vliet, Virginia. 1994. Apartheid and the politics of AIDS. In *Global AIDS Policy*, ed. Douglas A. Feldman. Westport, Connecticut: Bergin and Garvey, pp. 107–128.

Vis, Henri-L., Phillippe Hennart and Migabo Ruchababisha. 1981. Some issues in breast-feeding in deprived rural areas. *Assignment Children* 55/56: 183–200.

Wawer, Maria J., et al. 1997. Trends in HIV-1 prevalence may not reflect trends in incidence in mature epidemics: Data from the Raki population-based cohort, Uganda. *AIDS* 11: 1023–1030.

Widy-Wirski, R., et al. 1988. Evaluation of the WHO clinical case definition for AIDS in Uganda. *Journal of the American Medical Association* 260: 3286–3289.

Williams, C. D. 1938. Child health in the Gold Coast. *Lancet* 1: 97–102.

Winikoff, Beverly, Mary Ann Castle and Virginia Hight Laukaran, eds. 1988. *Feeding Infants in Four Societies*. New York: Greenwood Press.

World Health Organization. 1981. *International Code of Marketing of Breast-milk Substitutes*. Geneva, Switzerland: World Health Organization.

_____. 1989. *Weekly Epidemiological Record* 64: 42.

# PART THREE:

---

# *Politics and the Protection of Breastfeeding*

CHAPTER SIX

# The Political Momentum Following the International Code and the Nestlé Boycott

Decades of adversarial relations between the international agencies supporting breastfeeding and the formula manufacturers set a volatile political stage onto which the AIDS virus entered. For the agencies, the Nestlé boycott and the WHO Code were part of an established pattern of protecting breastfeeding.

## *Deadly Bottle-Feeding*

Initially, all mothers breastfed. But they long ago began to give their babies other liquids and semisolids. When baby bottles became available in local shops in resource-poor countries, mothers began to use them. The world seemed largely uninterested in how mothers fed their infants, until a few physicians began to describe some disastrous results. In 1939, Dr. Cicely Williams made an impassioned speech, called "Milk and Murder," to the Singapore Rotary Club. In it she focused attention on the marketing practices of the for-profit companies:

> If you are legal purists you may wish me to change the title of this address to Milk and Manslaughter. But if your lives were embittered as mine is, by seeing day after day this massacre of the innocents by

unsuitable feeding, then I believe you would feel as I do that mis-
guided propaganda on infant feeding should be punished as the most
miserable form of sedition, and that these deaths should be regarded
as murder.... Anyone who, ignorantly or lightly, causes a baby to be
fed on unsuitable milk, may be guilty of that child's death.

Williams also complained that the well-to-do women of Singapore aban-
doned breastfeeding because they wished to be free to go out and play
mahjong, or because they considered it beneath their dignity to feed their own
babies. What particularly distressed Williams was the marketing of sweetened
condensed milk as an infant food. Because it is deficient in vitamins, babies
who consumed it had gone blind from the lack of vitamin A and developed
rickets from the lack of vitamin D.

## The Free Powdered Milk

Another widespread example of bottle-feeding also involved something
other than infant formula. Shortly after UNICEF was created in 1946, it focused
efforts on remedying the rampant malnutrition seen in children at the end of
World War II. People then believed that protein deprivation was a major part
of malnutrition. This was at the same time that the United States government
announced it would donate powdered skim milk at no cost. The organization
distributed many thousands of tons of dried skim milk. Only in the early
years, however, was distribution of powdered milk a major part of UNICEF's
program (Teply 1979). Later UNICEF stopped the practice.

One big problem was that some of the powdered milk was ending up in
baby bottles, even though this had never been the intention of the program.
Jelliffe and Jelliffe (1978:234) noted that, with the knowledge of hindsight, it
had been a nutritional tragedy for well-intentioned programs to distribute
powdered milk: "As far as mothers of young children were concerned, this can
only have appeared as an endorsement of bottle-feeding, with a resulting dis-
placement effect on breast-feeding." Only women who had money could have
bought the totally inappropriate canned milk products that Dr. Williams complained of in 1939. But the powdered milk that UNICEF and other groups distributed was free.

UNICEF's later energetic promotion of breastfeeding was described as
being "part of undoing its own terrible mistake made in the name of nutrition" (Palmer 1993:226). That terrible mistake was distributing literally thousands of tons of powdered milk. The formula company marketing campaigns
followed all over the developing world where UNICEF and other charities had
helped "map out the roads" (Palmer 1993:227).

As years went on, formula companies increased their marketing activities until even little shops in developing countries sold infant formula. In a 1974 report from a World Food Conference, Blythe wrote,

> Lacking the money to buy substitute milk in the right quantities, impoverished parents "economize" by purchasing less and making it last longer. Medical workers have found that in some areas canned milk is being diluted up to three times the recommended amount. Exhortations to "sterilize bottles for ten minutes in clean boiling water" or to "keep your unopened baby-foods in the fridge" are meaningless to people who cannot read, who cook on hot embers, and have only seen refrigerators on advertising boardings in the towns. On such a grossly inadequate diet millions of babies lose weight, exhibit symptoms of marasmus and die before the age of six months. Those who are not killed outright by wasting away become vulnerable to infection.

The Jelliffes also noted that the availability of canned products and baby bottles accelerated the trend away from breastfeeding. They reasoned that women wanted breastmilk substitutes because they felt that these allowed them more freedom to work, and freedom from worry about the quantity or quality of their breastmilk. Like Coca-Cola, canned products had the appeal of being modern and Western. First the women of the elite classes chose to bottle-feed, and then other women wanted to do the same.

Companies marketed formula, cereals, and baby bottles in ways that encouraged women in developing countries to think that their babies would be better off with these products. Their ads reinforced any natural doubts mothers harbored about having enough milk. Many breastfeeding mothers believed, erroneously, that their babies would grow better if they also received formula.

Although more than thirty companies have been criticized for marketing their products, one word stands out in public consciousness: Nestlé. The giant Swiss food company is the largest formula producer and has been most accused of marketing its formulas all over the developing world. Those who organized a boycott decided to target Nestlé to concentrate their effectiveness, although the other formula companies were conducting similar activities (Barrington-Ward 1997).

## The 1970s and the Nestlé Boycott

In marketing their products, formula companies paid for jingles on local radio stations, ran pictures on billboards and posters showing fat happy (presumably bottle-fed) babies. Many labels on formula cans also had pictures of fat happy babies, though the feeding instructions may have been in a language that the mothers did not read. Formula companies used pictures of white doctors surrounded by black or Asian babies to give the idea that formula feeding was a modern healthy "first world" practice (Barrington-Ward 1997).

Many health workers went along with the policy of giving free formula to new mothers. Women dressed as "milk nurses" were allowed to give free formula to new mothers. After the free formula supply was used up, the mothers' breastmilk would have dried up, disallowing breastfeeding. Suckling would have triggered their bodies to start making milk again. But mothers generally did not realize that they could build up their milk supply by breastfeeding. Instead they were more likely to feed whatever they could afford.

In resource-poor countries, the price of formula is, given the average household income, exorbitant. A 1992 calculation compared the cost of formula for a three-month-old infant with the daily wage of a low-income worker, a hospital cleaner. An African family would have to spend 27–900 percent of their income to buy adequate amounts of formula at store prices (Cutting 1994).

Because they could not afford a full supply, women over-diluted the formula to make it go farther. They often used the only water available, which may have come from a polluted source, since bacterial contamination was common. No one taught them to boil water, or how to measure formula for proper reconstitution. If it looked milky, it seemed adequate for feeding. Babies became so malnourished and weakened that they could no longer fight off the diarrheal diseases and respiratory infections they encountered. Millions of babies died; millions more are dying.

In the early 1970s, groups in Europe published pamphlets accusing Nestlé of killing babies. Activists in many countries spread the word, and, by 1979, people in many countries began to boycott Nestlé products. The boycott has been described as one of the most successful grassroots political movements ever established.

Nestlé sued a small German group for criminal libel over the boycott campaign's defamatory title, "Nestlé Kills Babies." Nestlé won the lawsuit, although the fine was a token amount. The judge emphasized that the verdict did not exculpate Nestlé and told the company "to reconsider its advertising policies to avoid being accused of immoral conduct" (Infant-Food Industry 1976). Nestlé agreed and the boycott was officially ended in 1984, although it has since been revived in some countries. Many groups and individuals never stopped boycotting.

Other formula companies have been targeted in specific actions. For example, an order of nuns, the Sisters of the Precious Blood, sued Bristol-Myers (parent company of Mead-Johnson) to learn more about its marketing practices with infant formulas in "chronically impoverished third-world countries" (Infant Food Industry 1976). The case was dismissed, but the action had the desired effect of increasing public awareness of inappropriate marketing practices.

Consumer groups and individuals, at a 1979 meeting organized by the World Health Organization and UNICEF, launched the International Baby Food Action Network (IBFAN) to more effectively monitor the formula companies. IBFAN is made up of more than 140 groups in 70 countries. Small organizations like the Baby Milk Action Coalition in England and Canada's Infant Formula Action Coalition work cooperatively. The network has been very influential in calling attention to the issues surrounding the marketing practices of infant formula manufacturers.

Van Esterik noted that the need not to offend Western bottle-feeding families shaped the focus of the IBFAN groups. Recognizing that people in churches and women's groups might feel defensive about not breastfeeding their children at all, and be less likely to support a breastfeeding advocacy movement, the organizations downplayed the touchy and emotion-charged issue of how Westerners fed their babies. Little attention was focused on infant feeding decisions by individual mothers (Van Esterik 1989:105). Better, they concluded, to focus less on "breast is best" and more on "Nestlé is worst."

## The 1980s and the International Code

In May 1981, the World Health Assembly passed the International Code of Marketing of Breastmilk Substitutes. The assembly is the policy setting body of the World Health Organization, where representatives of all countries come together once a year. The passage of the Code came after a decade of intense work by activists and was an enormously important event. The Code was not designed to prohibit the sale of formula, but rather to set down rules for its ethical marketing and the marketing of bottles and rubber nipples or teats. It asked governments to protect and encourage breastfeeding, and it implored the companies to end promotion activities.

The 1981 Code was subsequently strengthened by resolutions in 1982, 1984, 1986, 1988, 1990, 1992, 1994, and 1996 and now contains guidelines for the ethical marketing of all types of breastmilk substitutes and calls for an end to their free distribution. These include formula for young babies, "follow up" formula for older babies, gruels, teas, juices and all other infant foods. The Code also applies to baby bottles, nipples (teats) and related equipment, calling for an end to advertising of all these products for babies.

The Code notes that health workers should not be pressured to accept gifts or funding for professional training in infant or child health or other financial inducements from companies whose products fall within its scope. It requires labels on formula and other foods for babies to be free of pictures. Labels, instead, should note the benefits of breastfeeding, the health hazards associated with improper use of foods such as formula, the negative effect of partial breastfeeding, and the difficulty in reversing the decision not to breastfeed.

## Violations to the Code Continue

Some extremely common practices are violations of the Code. Companies advertise baby bottles; give out posters, calendars, and pens to health workers; supply free formula to hospitals in some countries; and advertise their "follow up" formulas for older babies — all violations of the Code. The picture of the Gerber baby on a label is a violation of the Code, because she looks younger than four months.

Specific violations have been reported in recent years. One incident involved AIDS. In 1989 a representative of Nestlé was tape-recorded telling children in the United Kingdom that if HIV-positive mothers breastfeed, their babies run the risk of getting AIDS (Nestlé Accused 1989). He exaggerated the seroprevalence, which he said was "up to about 50 percent," whereas the prevalence among childbearing women had been only 30 percent in Kigali, Rwanda, in 1986 (Bizmungu 1989). He also said the HIV-positive mothers in African countries should not breastfeed, which at that time contradicted the existing WHO guidelines.

In 1993 protestors from IBFAN and the British group Baby Milk Action picketed a Nestlé shareholders' meeting. They wanted to show that they object to Nestlé giving free formula to some hospitals and promoting its products to health workers (Dillner 1993). IBFAN criticized Nestlé for organizing a cruise with the Brazilian Pediatric Society and allowing Brazilian physicians to go along for free. Nestlé Philippines was criticized for holding a raffle in a children's hospital and giving gifts to health workers.

Industry representatives have said that they want to have the boycott ended and that they will comply with the Code in resource-poor countries. As a result, the International Association of Infant Food Manufacturers (IFM), which represents the major baby food companies and all formula companies except Abbott/Ross and Bristol-Myers/Mead-Johnson, was accepted into official relations with the World Health Organization. But activists feel that as long as companies fail to comply, the boycott and the monitoring should continue and violations should be reported to the International Code Documentation Centre in Penang, Malaysia.

## The Slanging Match

While some groups continued to boycott, others, such as the Royal College of Midwives, decided that because the worst violations had stopped, protest was no longer warranted. No longer do the formula companies pay "milk nurses" to entice new mothers into bottle-feeding. Nor do companies give away free formula or baby foods in most countries.

In 1994 the Church of England "called for a hiatus in the slanging match between the manufacturers and IBFAN" (Barrington-Ward 1997). The Church, seeking to obtain independent research into the state of company marketing practices, joined with others in creating a new group, the Interagency Group on Breastfeeding Monitoring (IGBM). The research was coordinated from London and involved 27 churches, academic institutions and international nongovernmental organizations. The IGBM issued a report, called *Cracking The Code* (Interagency Group 1997), based on interviews with 800 pregnant women and new mothers, and 120 health workers in 40 facilities in Poland, Bangladesh, Thailand and South Africa.

*Cracking the Code* noted that the companies were still violating parts of the Code. Some formula company personnel, for instance, visited health care facilities uninvited and gave mothers printed information about their products. Other companies were found distributing printed materials and posters that displayed pictures of babies and occasionally brand names of formula.

Two of the four countries reported on — Thailand and South Africa — have very high rates of HIV. It may be that those who organized the monitoring for *Cracking the Code* were looking especially for HIV-related marketing practices when they selected these two countries out of the possible 190 that are monitored. The report did not acknowledge any HIV-related advertising schemes; in fact, it didn't mention HIV.

*Cracking the Code* (1997:14) reported, "There was no evidence from health workers' questionnaires of free or low-cost supplies of formula being provided in Bangladesh, Poland or South Africa." But 35 percent of the health care facilities in Thailand accepted free or low-cost supplies of formula and gave it to mothers. The report also failed to mention that the Thai government purchases formula and gives it away for free to babies of HIV-positive mothers who cannot afford to buy it. Noting that free formula was being given to 25 percent of hospitalized mothers in Thailand, which is more than the percentage who are HIV-positive, UNICEF concluded that hospitals did not limit free formula to HIV-positive mothers.

## Code Violations of 1997–1998

The publication of *Cracking the Code* was followed the next year by the publication of *Breaking the Rules, Stretching the Rules 1998* (IBFAN Penang 1998). The violations cited included donations of pens, prescription pads, tote bags, growth charts, posters, calendars, and clocks. Donations were made to support hospital-sponsored conferences, seminars and meetings. Health professionals attending scientific conferences were reimbursed for expenses. Formula companies violated the Code by having bunnies and teddy bears or occasionally pictures of babies on their labels. A number of companies omitted information from their label about the difficulty in reversing the decision not to breastfeed. Others gave mothers product information or a free sample. A Thai manufacturer was accused of breaking the Code by advertising baby bottles and a steam sterilizer.

*Breaking the Rules, Stretching the Rules* also criticized some companies for marketing water for babies. The company Humana, for instance, in advertising its Baby Wasser to parents, "violates the Code in several ways, not the least by its very name, inferring that cows' milk or water could be humanized (IBFAN Penang 1998:36). Nestlé was criticized for introducing two brands of water. One was found to have lower-than-average mineral content. The Swiss company was also criticized for developing a low-priced water for distribution in the Third World (IBFAN Penang 1998:36).

## Funding from Formula Companies

According to the World Health Organization, since the adoption of the Code, "the bulk of promotion budgets for infant formula has gone into providing gifts and other incentives to health professionals and institutions in the form of donated supplies, equipment, travel grants, etc." (Saadeh 1993:89). While some groups such as the Indian Academy of Paediatrics reject all such funding, the American Academy of Pediatrics, the Canadian Pediatric Association and the British Paediatric Association accept the money. UNICEF accepts money from Nestlé (First International Colloquium on Training 1996). The World Health Organization also accepts money from Nestlé, although a WHO representative noted that the organization does not use the Nestlé money for its infant nutrition programs (Saadeh 1997).

## Breastfeeding Activities in High Gear

The Code achieved the political momentum that enabled the World Health Organization and UNICEF to launch a global crusade for breastfeeding promotion. When the first reports about HIV transmission through breastfeeding appeared in the mid–1980s, the World Health Organization, and especially UNICEF, had already made breastfeeding a major focus of programs to foster child survival. UNICEF has, in many countries, conducted courses that train health workers to teach and encourage breastfeeding. For example, in 1994 UNICEF trained 217 people in Guinea-Bissau. Of the 217, 122 were trained in the promotion of breastfeeding. UNICEF funded radio and television programs promoting breastfeeding and immunization in many countries. In Guinea-Bissau, for example, breastfeeding and immunizations were the focus of at least two radio broadcasts daily for a year and one daily television spot for six months (UNICEF 1995).

UNICEF's current breastfeeding focus is the Baby Friendly Hospital Initiative. This hospital-based enterprise prohibits free formula and includes ten steps that hospitals need to follow to be designated "Baby Friendly." The goal of the initiative is to eliminate barriers to the smooth initiation of breastfeeding. Mothers who enter a hospital wanting to breastfeed should not encounter practices that make early breastfeeding difficult. They should not, for instance, have to wait hours to nurse their babies or have to deal with staff who do not understand breastfeeding. Neither should mothers have to try to breastfeed babies who have been bottle-fed or have to go home without any source of ongoing breastfeeding support.

Women who deliver in a Baby Friendly hospital are not required to breastfeed, but bottle-feeding mothers will be managed by the same rules. That means that all mothers (breast or bottle-feeding, cesarean or vaginal) will keep their babies in their rooms with them. Mothers are not to have their babies cared for in hospital nurseries, day or night. Nor will babies (breast or bottle-fed) be given pacifiers, although it was recently reported that bottle-fed babies who are put to bed with a pacifier have the risk of SIDS (crib death) reduced twentyfold (L'Hoir 1998).

In a highly unusual gesture, that made evident its commitment to the Baby Friendly Hospital Initiative, UNICEF gave money to a group in the United States to establish the United States Baby Friendly Initiative. Ordinarily, the only function of a national UNICEF committee in an industrialized country is to raise money. According to a UNICEF report, "The sole recipients of funds raised by National Committees are the children of the resource-poor world" (Bellamy 1996:68). Not so with Baby Friendly.

Unfortunately mothers may not follow the strong policies of some hospitals after they leave. A 1998 commentary from Zimbabwe noted that the pediatricians "who are realistic about what happens in the 'real world' know that sometimes these babies get bottles going home in the car, but in the hospital they breastfeed or they don't eat at all" (Morrison 1998). Szallasi (1998) noted that an accredited Australian Baby Friendly hospital had statistics showing a considerable drop off in breastfeeding rates early on. The reason given by the women for ceasing breastfeeding — "by an enormous margin" — was that they "don't like breastfeeding."

## A Unifying Concept for Breastfeeding

If there is one concept that pulls together all the political aspects of contemporary breastfeeding, it is the concept of protect-promote-support breastfeeding. In 1982, Dr. Ted Greiner first suggested the "protect-promote-support" framework that has been accepted in breastfeeding circles, pointing out that breastfeeding activities fall into three categories. *Protection* of breastfeeding refers to policies such as laws that make it illegal to sell formula or baby bottles without a prescription, and activities that guard women from forces that would lead them not to breastfeed. *Promotion* of breastfeeding seeks to convince reluctant women to breastfeed. Advertising is one way to promote breastfeeding. One drawback to promotion is that it can put undue pressure on women whose circumstances make exclusive breastfeeding difficult. Also, promotion often costs money, and after promotional activities are suspended, much of the positive effect may be lost. The major breast-feeding promotion campaign in Brazil increased breastfeeding rates. But after the media campaign and other outreach activities were cut back and then suspended, "breastfeeding prevalence and duration declined almost to the pre-campaign levels" (Green 1989). An evaluation of breastfeeding promotion efforts in Baltimore, Maryland, showed that the weak positive impact was largely gone by 7–10 days (Caulfield 1998). *Support* of breastfeeding involves activities that give breastfeeding mothers encouragement to keep breastfeeding. Women traditionally provided support for newly breastfeeding mothers. In industrialized countries breastfeeding support groups such as La Leche League provide mother-to-mother support. Labor-intensive activities such as home visits also support breastfeeding.

Greiner's (1993) central point was that it is inappropriate to promote breastfeeding until after protection and support activities are in place. While his main point may have become overshadowed, people seized upon his dictum that protective actions deserve high priority and are least likely to do harm (Greiner 1994). It has been argued that when funding and human resources are limited (as they always are in public health) one has to prioritize. Putting the emphasis on protection (as opposed to support or promotion) was seen as efficient and cost effective.

## AIDS Challenges Breastfeeding Protectionism

When the Nestlé boycott and the Code were instituted to protect breast-feeding, it seemed unimaginable that breastmilk would become potentially fatal for large numbers of babies. But protective policies in the most remote areas of the world are being changed by HIV/AIDS. Staff at a hospital in Western Samoa used to see no need to have any infant formula on hand. Whenever babies needed milk beyond what their mothers could provide, other mothers donated their extra breastmilk. Then came the report of two local mothers who were HIV-infected. One case involved a mother who died from AIDS though she had not been diagnosed with HIV. The other case involved a child who developed AIDS, which was the first indication that his mother was HIV-infected. No one knows if either of these mothers had donated (raw) breastmilk for other mothers' babies. Once it was recognized that

HIV was present in the population, the policy of giving babies other women's breastmilk was discontinued in favor of cup-feeding formula (Quested 1996).

HIV has also been reported in Papua New Guinea, an island nation in the South Pacific, just north of Australia. Papua New Guinea had originally tried to halt the decline in breastfeeding in 1976 when it banned all advertisements for bottle-feeding and mounted an educational campaign for health workers, community organizations and schools about the dangers of "artificial baby milk" (i.e., formula). But by the end of the year, it was clear that this not been at all effective. UNICEF noted, "It was clear that the battle was being lost. Sales of artificial baby milk were hardly affected and the attempt to persuade shop-keepers and supermarket chains to voluntarily restrict sales of feeding-bottles had had little or no effect" (Grant 1984:4).

After education failed to convince women to avoid bottle-feeding, Papua New Guinea passed a law in 1977 making the sale of baby bottles and nipples (teats) and pacifiers (dummies) prescription-only items. Health workers who did not follow the instructions in the law were liable for very stiff fines. Almost overnight, baby bottles disappeared from the shelves of shops. Bottle-feeding declined from 35 percent of the babies before the law was passed, to only 12 percent. Forty-seven percent of the bottle-feeding mothers worked away from home. The rate of gastroenteritis declined after bottles were restricted. Gastrointestinal deaths in babies under 6 months of age declined from three per year to one per year (Biddulph 1988).

Bottle-feeding now seems to be increasing, as satellite television beams in images of bottle-fed babies. Bottle-feeding is likely to further increase because HIV is increasing rapidly in Papua New Guinea, and as Health Minister Ludger Mond reported, 90 percent of new infections were among girls between the ages of 15 and 25 (Papua New Guinea 1997).

## The Code and HIV policy

Since the Code allows the use of formula or bottles, it is compatible with allowing HIV-infected mothers to choose alternatives to breastfeeding. Some people feel that HIV calls for no adaptation to the Code. Others feel that the Code should be amended to reflect the fact that HIV-positive mothers have a medical indication for formula.

The UNAIDS/WHO/UNICEF 1996–1997 statements about HIV and infant feeding remind manufacturers of their responsibilities under the Code. These include providing no free or low-cost supplies of formula, appropriate labeling, and no sponsorship of professional meetings. The 1994 World Health Assembly resolution, which reaffirmed the Code, addressed the issue of relief efforts. In emergency relief operations, donated supplies of breastmilk substitutes should be given only if they are continued for as long as infants need them, and supplies of donated substitutes should not be used as a sales inducement.

Representatives of the infant formula industry have said that they are ready to discuss with representatives of the World Health Organization the possibility of supplying formula as some form of relief effort (Meier 1997). In 1998 the Infant Food Manufacturers (IFM) was asked to work with UNICEF to supply formula for a ten-country demonstration project. Formula manufacturers are likely to be asked to make more formula available at or below cost for babies, in addition to the small numbers in the demonstration projects.

Walraven, Nicoll, Njau and Timaeus (1996) commented that there is a risk of lethal bottle-feeding in some areas after the risk of HIV infection through breastfeeding becomes widely known. They note that the situation "requires urgent but careful preparation and education of professionals and public alike." If the information is not presented carefully, the African cities could be a major battleground for breast versus bottle-feeding. The arena of the Nestlé boycott and the Code has long been emotion-charged and intensely political, and now, with the emergence of AIDS, it is likely to become even more fulminant. The battleground could well extend beyond the African cities.

# References

Baby Milk Action. 1997. HIV and infant feeding. *Baby Milk Action Update 21*, October.

Barrington-Ward, S. 1997. Putting babies before business. In *The Progress of Nations 1997: Nutrition Commentary*. New York: UNICEF, pp. 15–21.

Bellamy, Carol. 1996. *The State of the World's Children*. New York: UNICEF.

Biddulph, John. 1988. The Papua New Guinea programme. In *Programmes to Promote Breastfeeding*, eds. Derrick B. Jelliffe and E. F. Patrice Jelliffe. Oxford: Oxford University Press, pp. 161–165.

Bizmungu, C., et al. 1989. Nationwide community-based serological survey of HIV-1 and other human retrovirus infections. *Lancet* 335: 941–943.

Blythe, C. 1974. The great baby food scandal. *PAN* (Newspaper of the World Food Conference) No. 9, November 14.

Carballo, Manuel. 1988. The World Health Organization's work in the area of infant and young child feeding and nutrition. In *Programmes to Promote Breastfeeding*, eds. Derrick B. Jelliffe and E. F. Patrice Jelliffe. Oxford: Oxford University Press, pp. 235–247.

Caulfield, Laura E., et al. 1998. WIC-based interventions to promote breastfeeding among African-American women in Baltimore: Effects on breastfeeding initiation and continuation. *Journal of Human Lactation* 14: 15–22.

Cutting, William A. M. 1994. Breastfeeding and HIV in African countries. *Lancet* 343: 362.

Dillner, Luisa. 1993. Coffins greet Nestlé shareholders. *British Medical Journal* 306: 1563–1564.

*First International Training Colloquium.* 1996. Bangkok, Thailand, November 25–29.

Grant, James P. 1984. *The State of the World's Children.* New York: UNICEF.

Green, Cynthia P. 1989. *Media Promotion of Breastfeeding: A Decade's Experience.* Washington, D.C.: Academy for Educational Development for the U.S. Agency for International Development.

Greiner, Ted. 1982. Infant feeding policy options for governments. Report to the USAID-funded Infant Feeding Study Consortium: Population Council, Cornell and Columbia Universities, November.

———. 1993. Infant and young child nutrition: A historic review from a communication perspective. Introduction to *Communication Strategies to Support Infant and Young Child Nutrition*, ed. Peggy Koniz-Booher. Cornell International Nutrition Monographs 24–25 (combined), pp. 7–15.

———. 1994. Sustained breastfeeding, complementation and care. Revised and condensed version of a "Focus Paper" for the Cornell UNICEF Expert Working Group Colloquium on Care and Nutrition for the Young Child, Aurora New York, 12–15 October.

International Baby Food Action Network, Penang. 1998. *Breaking the Rules, Stretching the Rules.* Penang, Malaysia: IBFAN Penang.

Infant-Food Industry. 1976. *Lancet* ii: 503.

Interagency Group on Breastfeeding Monitoring. 1997. *Cracking the Code.* London: IGBM.

International Code of Marketing of Breastmilk Substitutes. 1981. *World Health Assembly Resolution 34.22,* May.

Jelliffe, Derrick B., and E. F. Patrice Jelliffe. 1978. *Human Milk in the Modern World.* London: Oxford University Press.

Joint WHO/UNICEF Statement. 1989. *Protecting, Promoting and Supporting Breastfeeding.* Geneva, Switzerland: World Health Organization.

L'Hoir, Monique, et al. 1998. Risk and preventive factors for death in the Netherlands, a low-incidence country. *European Journal of Pediatrics* 157 (8): 681–688.

Machekanyange, Zorodzai. 1997. Zimbabwe: Is breast milk still best? *Africa Information Afrique.* Harare, Zimbabwe, September 8.

Meier, Barry. 1997. In war against AIDS, battle over baby formula reignites. *New York Times,* June 8, pp.1, 16.

Morrison, Pamela. 1998. *Guilt.* Available from lactnet@library.ummed.edu; INTERNET, June 18.

Nestlé accused of false AIDS claims. 1989. *Lancet* ii, November 25, p. 1289.

Palmer, Gabrielle. 1993. *The Politics of Breastfeeding.* London: Pandora Press.

Papua New Guinea Health Minister says AIDS reaching crisis level. 1997. *Reuters News Service,* August 22.

Quested, Christine. 1996. Personal communication at the Global Forum on Breastfeeding, Bangkok, Thailand, December 2–6.

Saadeh, Randa J., Miriam H. Labbok, Kristin A. Cooney and Peggy Koniz-Booher,

eds. 1993. *Breast-feeding: The Technical Basis for Action*. Geneva, Switzerland: World Health Organization.

Szallasi, Trudi. 1998. Why women wean. Available from lactnet@library.ummed.edu; INTERNET, June 15.

Teply, L. J. 1979. Breastfeeding, milk and UNICEF. In *Breastfeeding and Food Policy in a Hungry World*, ed. Dana Raphael. New York: Academic Press, pp. 253–258.

UNAIDS Joint United Nations Programme on HIV/AIDS. 1996. HIV and Infant Feeding: An Interim Statement. *Weekly Epidemiological Record* 71: 289–291.

UNICEF. 1995. *Selected examples of UNICEF input in 1994*. New York: UNICEF. (Also available at http://www.unicef.org; INTERNET.)

_____. 1996. *Fifty Years for Children*. New York: UNICEF.

Van Esterik, Penny. 1989. *Beyond the Breast-Bottle Controversy*. New Brunswick, New Jersey: Rutgers University Press.

Walraven, G., et al. 1996. The impact of HIV-1 infection on child health in sub–Saharan Africa: Burden on health services. *Tropical Medicine and International Health* 1: 3–14.

Williams, Cicely. 1939. *Milk and Murder: Address to Singapore Rotary Club*. Penang, Malaysia: International Organization of Consumers Unions.

CHAPTER SEVEN

# For Breastfeeding, Too, the Band Played On

In 1987 Randy Shilts' book *And the Band Played On* was first published. Shilts, who later died of AIDS, was the San Francisco reporter who documented what was happening during the early years of the AIDS epidemic. He described the story of the politics and the people, and the way in which the most trusted institutions downplayed the threat of AIDS. This chapter follows Shilts' example in chronicling how leading international health agencies and others downplayed the role of breastmilk in transmitting HIV.

In 1997 a physician who hosts a weekly live Internet conference about international pediatrics expressed his shock at reading an article in the *New York Times* about breastfeeding and AIDS. Dr. Julius Edlavitch noted that Barry Meier's article about AIDS and breastmilk raised some incredible issues: "Anyone who dedicates themselves to increasing breastfeeding amongst the developing countries must be very stressed over the findings in this article."

But why didn't a physician who is dedicated to international breastfeeding know about HIV and breastfeeding before a newspaper reported it? Edlavitch's reaction implies that whatever publications he had been following for the past ten years had failed to call his attention to the HIV-breastfeeding research published in the prestigious peer-reviewed medical journals.

Clearly Edlavitch was not the only person who had not been informed about HIV and breastfeeding. African delegates to the May 1997 World Health Assembly expressed their unhappiness at not being given needed information. The delegate from Lesotho noted that member states of the UN had not been provided with clear guidance about how HIV-infected women might best feed their babies (Turmen 1997). Zimbabwe's Health and Child Welfare Minister Timothy Stamps (1997) also noted that the international health agencies had not been keeping the African ministers of health apprised about breastfeeding and HIV. Stamps presented a common submission at the World Health Assembly on behalf of Angola, Botswana, Lesotho, Malawi, Mauritius, and South Africa. He criticized UNICEF and the World Health Organization for not devising helpful interventions: "Are we to accept that our children's survival should be compromised by the risk of infant AIDS in the cruelest sense through the promotion of unlimited, unmodified and unchallenged breast-feeding policies?"

## Not Talking About HIV

Greiner, who had conceptualized the protect-promote-support model for breastfeeding, feared that the formula companies might spread information about HIV and breastfeeding. In a talk to the Bangladeshi Breastfeeding Foundation, Greiner's recommendation was to ask the companies "not to talk about it in public" (Greiner 1997). Greiner's phrase "not to talk about it" seems like a succinct description of the modus operandi. Edlavitch, Stamps and others who were very familiar with breastfeeding might have been more familiar with HIV if the information had been passed along to them. But either the primary research articles about HIV and breastfeeding were not discussed, or the findings were given a better spin when they were mentioned in secondary sources. Looking back now at some of the reports from the 1980s and 1990s gives an overview of what the international agencies were saying about breastfeeding and about HIV. Annually published reports such as UNICEF's *State of the World's Children* are particularly revealing.

The 1981-1982 *State of the World's Children* announced the International Code of Marketing of Breastmilk Substitutes, which the World Health Assembly passed overwhelmingly in May 1981; only the United States had voted against it. This was just one month before the CDC first reported that a few gay men had an opportunistic infection later noted to be associated with AIDS. No connection between breastfeeding and an unusual pneumonia in gay men seemed imaginable.

In the 1982-1983 *State of the World's Children*, Executive Director James Grant announced "a children's revolution." Breastfeeding was to be one-fourth of a children's survival revolution, one-fourth of a world revolution being a huge undertaking. The four specific techniques to improve infant and child mortality rates were referred to as GOBI: *g*rowth monitoring, *o*ral rehydration therapy, *b*reastfeeding and *i*mmunizations.

The legacy of GOBI is still in place. UNAIDS' Director Peter Piot noted some of his experiences: "In Africa, in Asia, in many places that I travel, I see volunteers going door to door to make sure that every child turns up for the next vaccination, or to support new mothers in breastfeeding, or to explain how to use ORT [oral rehydration therapy]" (Piot 1997).

The 1984 *State of the World's Children* report also noted that the four activities, including breastfeeding, occupied a special place. But the 1985 report was more cautious. It noted that the next few years would tell if breastfeeding promotion could succeed in halting the march of bottle-feeding. In the 1986 and 1987 editions there was less talk about breastfeeding. Oral rehydration and immunizations received much more attention, although UNICEF did not explain why. In 1983 breastfeeding had been one-fourth of a world child survival revolution, but it wasn't in 1987.

## Less Talk About Breastfeeding

UNICEF never explained why it placed less emphasis on breastfeeding between 1983 and 1987. In contrast to earlier editions of the *State of the World's Children* report, the 1987 report hardly mentioned breastfeeding. Van Esterik (1989:198) noted UNICEF's lessened interest in breastfeeding and suggested a reason why UNICEF might have placed less emphasis on breastfeeding and more on immunizations and oral rehydration solutions. The latter interventions are, she insists, more entrenched in the development industry and provide opportunities for pharmaceutical companies to make large profitable contracts.

Raphael (1994:135), on the other hand, observed that UNICEF began to de-emphasize breastfeeding just as HIV transmission through breastmilk was recognized in Western medical journals (Ziegler 1985, Thiry 1985, CDC 1985, Blanche 1986, Lepage 1987, Mok 1987, Senturia 1987). Nor was there much by way of solace in other scientific reports. Researchers already knew that maternal milk was a major mode of transmission for many animal retroviruses (Adams 1983, DeBoer 1979, Narayan 1985, Teich 1984). It was also known that breastmilk was a major mode of transmission for the first recognized human retrovirus, HTLV-I (Kinoshita 1984). Researchers, moreover, had already confirmed that HIV was a retrovirus. In the mid-to-late 1980s, some hoped that the antibodies in breastmilk would protect babies even though antibodies generally did not stop milk-borne transmission of other retroviruses. Also, by the end of 1986, people realized the magnitude of the epidemic in Africa (Barnett and Blaikie 1992:1). In short, there was good reason to worry.

If UNICEF's strongest promotion of breastfeeding slacked off between 1983 and 1987, this is understandable. Those who had the benefit of scientific advisors must have recognized that HIV transmission via breastmilk was a potentially huge problem. Although UNICEF has continued to promote breastfeeding, the emphasis has lessened.

If there was any doubt that HIV/AIDS could devastate breastfeeding programs, it was soon shattered with the early reports from Africa. Take for example the scene in 1988. The report had just come in from Kinshasa, capital city of Zaire (now renamed Democratic Republic of Congo). A radio broadcaster pointed out the connection between breastfeeding and AIDS. There was an immediate 30 percent drop in breastfeeding initiation rates (Greiner 1997). That 30 percent drop must have been the most unwelcome news to those who were trying to restore exclusive breastfeeding. And this was just one of many radio reports in Africa, where people get much of their news from radio and word of mouth.

Barnett and Blaikie (1992:105–106) noted that Ugandan women suspend the urgency of other activities at the markets, church and roadside to listen and talk to one another. In their conversations, women discuss, among other things, AIDS and feeding babies.

## HIV as a Threat to Breastfeeding

In 1987 the World Health Organization issued a statement about HIV and infant feeding. It noted that there was insufficient evidence to conclude that breastfeeding was a significant source of HIV transmission, and that in developing countries, breastfeeding was a lifesaving intervention.

AIDS researchers Le Coeur and Lallemant (1996:275) suggested a reason for the 1987 World Health Organization position:

> New doubts about the safety of breast-feeding related to HIV infection were seen by many public health agencies as a threat to years of prevention efforts. Accordingly, the position initially adopted in 1987 by the World Health Organization for developing countries was conservative: despite the expansion of the HIV epidemic among women of child-bearing age, breast-feeding was still recommended.

Dr. Susan E. Holck, an expert on breastfeeding at the World Health Organization, said that she was "struck by how much denial there was around 1990 of the evidence we had that HIV could be transmitted through breast-feeding." Much of the denial, she claimed, "undoubtedly was fed by people who had invested so much in promoting breastfeeding and feared what confirmation of that transmission might do to the gains that were made in breastfeeding" (Altman 1998).

Director of the Human Lactation Center Dr. Dana Raphael (1994:134–135) noted that humanitarian organizations such as UNICEF and the World Health Organization had downplayed the negative effect of HIV out of fear that it would devastate breastfeeding campaigns. She suggested that the international agencies were reluctant to give up the worldwide support for breastfeeding, which had become lucrative. "As so often happens when absolutes are challenged by new evidence, researchers were able to turn the findings of the potentially lethal effect of breast milk, confirmed by their own research, to accommodate the overall political needs and economic status of their agencies."

UNICEF's 1988 *State of the World's Children* report acknowledged that AIDS threatened breastfeeding: "AIDS could also pose an indirect threat to millions more children if misinformation about the disease is allowed to affect immunization and breastfeeding programmes" (Grant 1988:18).

This 1988 *State of the World's Children* report also claimed that it is theoretically possible that breastfeeding can transmit the AIDS virus and "worldwide there are two cases where this is thought to have happened." It is not clear which are the "two" cases acknowledged in this 1988 report, even if one counts only the reports already published in the medical journals (Ziegler 1985, Thiry 1985, Blanche 1986, Lepage 1987, Mok 1987, Senturia 1987, Friedland 1987, Minkoff 1987).

## Early 1990s: Not Talking About HIV

In August 1990 the major breastfeeding policy groups came together in Florence, Italy. In the years leading up to the meeting, more and more researchers were reporting HIV transmission through breastfeeding, and more African newspapers were carrying stories about breastfeeding and HIV. The meeting produced the Innocenti Declaration, which stressed the need to protect, promote and support breastfeeding. But the Innocenti Declaration never mentioned HIV/AIDS.

By contrast, the Pan American Health Organization (PAHO) convened a meeting in 1990 at which pediatricians and public health officers from throughout Latin America strongly endorsed the recommendation that HIV-positive women be advised to avoid breastfeeding (PAHO 1990). PAHO is an international public health agency with more than ninety years' experience and predates the World Health Organization, for which it now serves as the Regional Office of the Americas.

## Less and Less Talk About HIV and Breastfeeding

UNICEF's 1989, 1990 and 1991 *State of the World's Children* reports each had a full-page panel devoted to AIDS. The 1989 report insisted that "breastfeeding is not a significant means of transmitting AIDS," though it cited no research that corroborated its position. The Italian Multicenter Study (1988) had reported that HIV transmission rates were higher among children who were born by vaginal delivery and breastfed. Of the 65 Italian breastfed babies, 46 became HIV-infected.

In 1988 Van de Perre reported that of the four Rwandan women whose milk he studied, three had babies who were HIV-positive. In 1989 Hira reported that 39 percent of HIV-positive Zambian women had HIV-positive babies. In 1991 Van de Perre reported that 45–60 percent of children became HIV-infected if they were being breastfed at the time that their originally HIV-negative mothers seroconverted. In 1991 Hira also concluded that children of initially HIV-negative mothers risked infection following maternal seroconversion. Maternal HIV infections were presumed to have happened via sexual contacts.

UNICEF's 1990 and 1991 full-panel reports on AIDS simply omitted any reference to breastfeeding and AIDS. In 1992, UNICEF's *State of the World's Children* report had only one sentence about mother-to-child transmission; it stated that one million children have been "born HIV-positive."

Later *State of the World's Children* reports also failed to address the emerging picture of HIV transmission through breastfeeding, even though the medical journals and conferences were making significant announcements. The European Collaborative Study, for example, reported in 1991 that 32 percent of babies breastfed by HIV-positive mothers became infected, compared to 12 percent of bottle-fed babies.

In 1991 Baker reported that many women in Zambia knew that breastfeeding can transmit HIV and were afraid to breastfeed. Further, health workers in Zambia were accusing authorities of employing a double standard for infant feeding in developed and developing counties. UNICEF's 1992 *State of the World's Children* did not mention breastfeeding and HIV.

The 1992 WHO/UNICEF consensus statement recommended that women known to be HIV-infected continue to breastfeed, except for those who lived where infection and malnutrition were not major causes of infant death. Within days after the WHO issued a press release with these recommendations, a newspaper in Kenya carried the report with a story whose headline read, "HIV transmitted by breastfeeding" (Berer 1993).

In 1992, Dunn's meta-analysis received much attention because it was the first to quantify the risk of HIV transmission attributable to breastfeeding. But UNICEF's 1993 *State of the World's Children* report again failed to address HIV/AIDS. In 1993, UNICEF published a lengthy booklet entitled *AIDS: The Second Decade.* UNICEF Executive Director James Grant described in detail efforts to reduce HIV infections among adults and adolescents, but this report from a children's organization did not discuss how children become HIV-infected. The one relevant sentence in the long report fails to clarify the role of breastfeeding and HIV: "Approximately one of three children born to these women is HIV-infected."

In 1993, the World Health Organization published a book called *Breast-*

*feeding: The Technical Basis and Recommendations for Action.* The book referred
to discussions about research on the possible transmission of HIV through
breastmilk as belonging under the category of "spreading false rumors" (Saadeh
1993:87).

In 1993, Embree reported that 49 percent of Nairobi children breastfed
by HIV-infected mothers for at least 15 months became HIV-infected. In 1993,
Pitts and Jackson reported that AIDS was the most common cause of death in
children in major hospitals in Zimbabwe. In 1993, Kingman reported that HIV
caused nearly all deaths in people aged 13–39 in rural Uganda. UNICEF's 1994
*State of the World's Children* acknowledged that AIDS was reversing hard-won
gains in child mortality but never told readers how it is that children get AIDS.
It said that children are "born with the virus."

Some 1994 reports documented significant rates of HIV transmission
among breastfed babies in Congo (Lallemant), in Kenya (Datta), and in
Rwanda (Simonon). But UNICEF's 1995 *State of the World's Children* report
mentioned very briefly that HIV was known to have been transmitted in breastmilk in some instances.

In 1995, the Minister of Health of Swaziland reported that the majority
of babies admitted to the country's hospitals were treated for HIV-related illnesses (Swazi Babies 1995). In 1995, Al-Nozha reported that nine out of nine
Saudi Arabian babies breastfed by HIV-infected mothers became infected. In
similar studies, Kumar revealed that 48 percent of Indian babies breastfed by
HIV-infected mothers became infected, and Taha related that the rate was 35
percent in Malawi.

UNICEF's 1996 *State of the World's Children* report referred to HIV/AIDS
very briefly, noting only that children become orphaned when their parents
die of AIDS. The report never mentioned that children can become HIV-infected
by their mothers. The report also discussed the under–5 mortality rate (the
rate of child mortality for children up to their fifth birthday). It said that this
rate "appears to have increased in several countries, including Madagascar,
Zambia and Zimbabwe" (Bellamy 1996:46). It never said why.

UNICEF's 1996 *Promise and Progress: Achieving Goals for Children* also
noted that the under–5 mortality rates were up in some areas, largely in
sub–Saharan Africa and South Asia. Again, UNICEF did not explain why, but
recommended that the countries "adopt more realistic targets" for their
under–5 mortality rates (UNICEF 1996a).

## Newer Policies

In 1996 UNAIDS/WHO/UNICEF jointly issued an interim statement about
HIV and infant feeding, which the WHO (1996) published, and which became
a Policy Statement in 1997. It recommended informed choice, although UNAIDS

(1997a) later noted that, in most poor countries, most women are not provided with sufficient information and support to make an informed choice.

In 1996 Rubini reported that HIV transmission rates were more than double among breastfed babies, compared to bottle-fed babies. UNICEF's 1997 *State of the World's Children* report mentioned HIV/AIDS very briefly, and then only to note that the epidemic had pushed more children into the labor market because their parents died. Even though AIDS had become the leading cause of death for children in a growing number of countries, the report never mentioned AIDS in children.

UNAIDS (1997b) noted that, in Namibia, HIV caused nearly twice as many deaths across all ages as malaria, the next most common killer. In the trading centers of Uganda, nearly nine out of ten deaths are related to AIDS. A report issued in conjunction with the 1996 International Conference on AIDS suggested that AIDS may increase child mortality rates in Zambia nearly threefold by the year 2010 (Status and Trends 1996).

In 1997 the World Health Organization issued a fact sheet called "Reducing Mortality from Major Childhood Killer Diseases." It never mentioned HIV/AIDS. Even in the section about major childhood killer diseases in Zambia, AIDS was never mentioned, even though it is the leading cause of child death in Zambia. In that report, the WHO noted that when bottle-feeding increased between 1972 and 1992, infant mortality increased by 35 percent. The report, then, noted the 35 percent bottle-related increase, but did not mention the estimated 100–300 percent AIDS-related increase.

UNICEF's 1998 *State of the World's Children* report does have a section on breastmilk and transmission of HIV. It makes many of the same recommendations as UNAIDS, suggesting, for instance, that voluntary testing and counseling be made more accessible. It states that if an HIV-positive mother has access to adequate breastmilk substitutes that she can prepare safely, she should consider using them, wet-nursing or heat treatment of expressed breastmilk.

UNICEF and the WHO were not the only agencies whose breastfeeding policies were challenged by the threat of HIV/AIDS. The U.S. General Accounting Office (GAO) had strongly recommended to the Congress in 1993 that information about HIV be routinely given to all pregnant women participating in the government's Women, Infants and Children Program (WIC). The opportunity for education is enormous, since approximately one-half of all U.S. babies participate in the program. The GAO recommendation has yet to be implemented.

La Leche League International (1997) told readers through its media release that the extent to which HIV can be passed through breastmilk and the role of human milk in fighting HIV remain unclear: "Human milk may contain factors that prevent the binding of HIV to specific receptor sites on human cells. This phenomenon potentially inhibits the virus from taking hold in the baby."

## Commentaries

Various commentators have suggested reasons why pro-breastfeeding groups have reacted to HIV as they have. Nicholas Eberstadt, a researcher with the Harvard Center for Population and Development Studies, opined that UNICEF's "blinding ideology" to promoting breastfeeding and boycotting Nestlé had left it particularly ill equipped to deal with HIV transmission through breastfeeding: "You can think of UNICEF's medical obtuseness as a cruel manifestation of bureaucratic inefficiency, a product of blinding ideology, a simple human tragedy, or some combination of the three."

Elliott Abrams (1997), who had been U.S. Assistant Secretary of State for International Organizations, also accused UNICEF of being addicted to ideology and, in particular, to the belief that breast is always best. Abrams, in fact, went so far as to declare that UNICEF was in a state of denial.

Zambian gynecologist Mavis Sianga was critical of the fact that free formula is prohibited for babies of HIV-infected mothers: "It is rather unfair that women in developing countries must risk passing on the infection just because WHO and UNICEF want to keep their programs flying" (Geloo 1998). She feels that a policy of not helping HIV-infected women to formula-feed has chauvinistic overtones:

> We have condoms to protect us against AIDS, but the decision on use always lies with men. They decide if they want to protect themselves. The condoms are everywhere and cheap. Now, when it comes to a woman wanting to protect her baby, it is suddenly political, it is cultural, it is expensive, it is impossible. What nonsense is this? (Geloo 1998)

Women and AIDS Support Network coordinator Priscilla Misihairambwi noted the World Health Organization appears to have a double standard concerning breastfeeding and HIV transmission: "In the affluent, industrialized countries the WHO advises HIV-infected women to stop breastfeeding and give their children milk substitutes, while in developing countries HIV-infected women are advised to carry on breastfeeding." She argued that the WHO did not do its research on how Africans feed babies when mothers are unable to breastfeed, and that the WHO assumes that Africans cannot make decisions about their children's health (Machekanyange 1997). The debate over the use of placebos in perinatal AZT trials also led some researchers to say that they resent the debate's implications that Africans cannot decide what is best for themselves (French 1997).

Rita Gorna, chairperson of the Community Planning Committee of the 1998 International Conference on AIDS, suggested that the initial healthy skepticism about breastfeeding and HIV has dragged on too long, as conspiracy theories tend to overstay their welcome (Gorna 1996:241). People tend to acknowledge dangers only with activities that they want to see as risky. Because we do not want to see breastfeeding as risky, we are resistant.

Dr. Miriam Labbok of USAID has long promoted breastfeeding in the context of fertility control and LAM (Labbok 1981, 1983, 1984, 1985, 1989, 1991, 1994, 1997a). She concluded, "Most models, based on the current understanding of HIV transmission, support continued recommendation of breastfeeding for all women ... except in situations where a woman knows her HIV status is positive and where there is affordable availability of high quality breastmilk substitutes" (Labbok 1997b).

A 1997 report from a World Bank symposium implied that breastfeeding by HIV-infected women is almost praiseworthy. From the symposium "Breastfeeding and AIDS: The Tragedy Unfolds" comes this statement:

> The most noteworthy aspect of a recent Bank symposium ... was the unexpected agreement that, even in light of reports about mothers transmitting HIV via breast milk, breastfeeding by HIV-infected mothers should be encouraged.... If breastfeeding didn't exist and someone invented it ... the Nobel Committee would be forced to give two Nobel Prizes — one for medicine and one for economics. (Berg 1997)

The report, however, does not call for mothers to be surveyed regarding their feelings about the policy of encouraging HIV-infected women to breastfeed.

## Spring of 1998

On March 11, 1998, UNICEF announced its continued support of breastfeeding despite the possible risk of HIV transmission (Children: UNICEF Backs Breastfeeding 1998). But at a March 23–24, 1998, meeting, UNAIDS noted the evidence supporting the position that HIV-positive mothers not breastfeed and recommended that they be helped with access to safe alternatives. On March 26, 1998, UNICEF issued a press release stating that it would distribute infant formula:

> Infant formula, at affordable prices and in the quantity needed for about six months, for tested women with HIV who make an informed choice in favour of this alternative. Formula with no brand labels will be distributed at reduced cost through existing community-based institutions with careful control, targeting and monitoring.... UNICEF hopes to engage local and, if necessary, multinational manufacturers of dairy products, including infant formula, as partners in this effort, depending on their willingness to provide generically labeled quality formula that will not represent a commercial gain.

In April 1998 the WHO convened a three-day technical consultation to discuss HIV and infant feeding. At the meeting, documents about HIV and infant feeding were introduced. Dr. Ruth Nduati (1998) had prepared a review document in which she described the use of breastmilk substitutes as "a therapeutic intervention that should be prescribed and supported with health education on safe handling." She also noted that there was "lukewarm interest" in identifying ways to mobilize resources to support breastmilk substitutes. She speculated that a loss of confidence in the health care system might result if the problem of HIV transmission through breastfeeding continued to be ignored. This in turn can have a negative impact on other important health care interventions.

In addition to Dr. Nduati's review, other documents distributed at the WHO Technical Consultation included a set of guidelines for decision makers and a set of guidelines for health care managers and supervisors. The aim of the guidelines was not to recommend policies, but rather to discuss issues to be considered. Policy decisions need to be made by local authorities. The guidelines emphasize the importance of voluntary testing and counseling programs and of HIV-status awareness. They also stress the need to protect, promote and support breastfeeding: "In formulating policies to prevent HIV transmission through breastfeeding, care should be taken to prevent the 'spillover effect,' in which fear of HIV infection undermines the commitment to breastfeeding even among women who are not infected — and undermines too, support by health systems and policies for breastfeeding."

Those attending the May 1998 World Health Assembly noted that, prior to the convention, it had been decided to welcome new WHO director-general Dr. Gro Bruntland and to minimize discussion of the issue of breastfeeding and HIV.

## The Pace of Responses

The announcement that short-term use of AZT reduced mother-to-child HIV transmission in Thailand by 51 percent (Joint Statement) was followed one month later by an UNAIDS meeting (UNAIDS 1998). The aim was to take "concerted action" in response to the Thai results. Discussions about alternatives to breastfeeding, however, have proceeded at a much slower pace than a one-month turn around. The slower pace is clearly related to a desire to protect breastfeeding. But the public health goal of protecting breastfeeding and the slow pace of deliberations seem far removed from the thinking of the women involved.

# References

Abrams, Elliott. 1997. UNICEF is all trick and no treat. *Washington Times*, October 31.

Adams, D. S., et al. 1983. Transmission and control of caprine arthritis-encephalitis virus. *American Journal of Veterinary Research* 44: 1670–1675.

Al-Nozha, M. M., A. R. Al-Frath, M. Al-Nasser and S. Ramia. 1995. Horizontal versus vertical transmission of human immunodeficiency virus type 1 (HIV-1). *Tropical and Geographical Medicine* 47(6): 293–295.

Altman, Lawrence K. 1998. AIDS brings a shift on breastfeeding. *New York Times*, July 26, p. 1.

Baker, Kristi, and Vivien Nakawala. 1991. Breastfeeding and AIDS survey. *NGO AIDS Newsletter* (Family Health Trust, Lusaka): 2, April 4.

Barnett, Tony, and Piers Blaikie. 1992. *AIDS in Africa: Its Present and Future Impact*. New York: Guilford Press.

Bellamy, Carol. 1996. *The State of the World's Children*. New York: UNICEF.

_____. 1997. *The State of the World's Children*. New York: UNICEF.

_____. 1998. *The State of the World's Children*. New York: UNICEF.

Berer, Marge, with Sunanda Ray. 1993. *Women and HIV/AIDS*. London: Pandora Press.

Berg, Alan. 1997. Breast still best. *World Bank Office Memorandum: New & Noteworthy in Nutrition* 30: 8.

Blanche, S., et al. 1986. Infection à LAV et syndrome immunodéficitaire acquis (SIDA) chez le nourrisson. *Archives French Pediatrics* 43: 87–92.

_____, et al. 1989. A prospective study of perinatal infection of infants born to women seropositive for human immunodeficiency virus type 1. *New England Journal of Medicine* 320: 1643–1648.

Bobat, R., Moodley Dhayendree, Anna Coutsoudis and Hoosen Coovadia. 1997. Breastfeeding by HIV-1-infected women and outcome in their infants: A cohort study from Durban, South Africa. *AIDS* 11:1627–1633.

Carter, Pam. 1995. *Feminism, Breasts and Breast-Feeding*. New York: St. Martin's Press.

Centers for Disease Control and Prevention. 1985. Recommendations for assisting in the prevention of perinatal transmission of human T-lymphotropic virus type III/lymphaedeonopathy. *Morbidity and Mortality Weekly Report* 34: 721–732.

Children: UNICEF Backs Breastfeeding Over AIDS Threat. IPS *Wire*, March 11, 1998.

Datta, Pratibha, et al. 1994. Mother-to-child transmission of human immunodeficiency virus type 1: Report from the Nairobi study. *Journal of Infectious Diseases* 170: 1134–1140.

DeBoer, G. F., C. Terpstra, D. J. Houwers and J. Hendriks. 1979. Studies in epidemiology of Maedi visna in sheep. *Research in Veterinary Science* 26: 202–208.

Eberstadt, Nicholas. 1997. Trick and mistreat. *The New Republic*, November 10, pp. 13–14.

Edlavitch, Julius. 1997. *NY Times* article. Available from edlav001@maroon.tc.umn.edu; INTERNET, June 10.

Embree, J., et al. 1993. Delayed seroconversion in infants born to HIV-1 seropositive mothers: Associated factors. Presented at the Ninth International Conference on AIDS, Berlin, Germany, June 6–11. Abstract WS-CO2-4.

European Collaborative Study. 1991. Children born to women with HIV-1 infection: Natural history and risk of transmission. *Lancet* 337: 253–260.

French, Howard W. 1997. AIDS research in Africa: Juggling risks and hopes. *New York Times*, October 9, p. A1.

Friedland, G. H., and R. S. Klein. 1987. Transmission of human immunodeficiency virus. *New England Journal of Medicine* 317: 1125–1135.

Gabiano, C., et al. 1991. HIV-1 transmission rate in first born children to seropositive mothers and interfering factors. Presented at the Seventh International Conference on AIDS, Florence, Italy, June 16–21.

Geloo, Zarina. 1998. HIV and Breastfeeding: Reigniting an old controversy. Women's Feature Service. *Women's International Net Magazine*. Available at http://www.geocities.com/wellesley/3321/win6d.htm; INTERNET.

Global Programme on AIDS. 1992. Consensus statement from the WHO/UNICEF Constitution on HIV transmission and breast feeding. *Weekly Epidemiological Record* 67: 177–184.

Gorna, Robin. 1996. *Vamps, Virgins and Victims: How Women Can Fight AIDS*. London: Cassell, Wellington House.

Grant, James P. 1981-1982. *The State of the World's Children*. New York: UNICEF.
_____. 1982-1983. *The State of the World's Children*. New York: UNICEF.
_____. 1984. *The State of the World's Children*. New York: UNICEF.
_____. 1985. *The State of the World's Children*. New York: UNICEF.
_____. 1986. *The State of the World's Children*. New York: UNICEF.
_____. 1987. *The State of the World's Children*. New York: UNICEF.
_____. 1988a. UNICEF programmes in promotion of breastfeeding. In *Programmes to Promote Breastfeeding*, eds. Derrick B. Jelliffe and E. F. Patrice Jelliffe. Oxford: Oxford University Press, pp. 227–234.
_____. 1988b. *The State of the World's Children*. New York: UNICEF.
_____. 1989. *The State of the World's Children*. New York: UNICEF.
_____. 1990. *The State of the World's Children*. New York: UNICEF.
_____. 1991. *The State of the World's Children*. New York: UNICEF.
_____. 1992. *The State of the World's Children*. New York: UNICEF.
_____. 1993a. *AIDS: The Second Decade*. New York: UNICEF.
_____. 1993b. *The State of the World's Children*. New York: UNICEF.
_____. 1994. *The State of the World's Children*. New York: UNICEF.
_____. 1995. *The State of the World's Children*. New York: UNICEF.

Gray, Glenda E., J. A. McIntyre and S. F. Lyons. 1996. The effect of breastfeeding on vertical transmission of HIV-1 in Soweto, South Africa. Presented at the Eleventh International Conference on AIDS, Vancouver, Canada, July 7–12. Abstract Th.C.415.

Greiner, Ted. 1997. The HIV threat to breastfeeding: Virus, fear and greed. Modified from a talk to the Bangladeshi Breastfeeding Foundation, August 29.

Innocenti Declaration. 1991. On the protection, promotion and support of breastfeeding. *Ecology of Food and Nutrition* 26: 271–273.

Italian Multicentre Study. 1988. Epidemiology, clinical features, and prognostic factors of paediatric HIV infection. *Lancet* 2: 1043–1045.

Joint Statement by CDC, UNAIDS, NIH and ANRS. 1998. (Following the) Announcement by the Ministry of Public Health of Thailand and the CDC of Results from Their Mother-to-Child Transmission Trial, February 20.

Joint United Nations Programme on HIV/AIDS (UNAIDS). 1996. HIV and infant feeding: An interim statement. *Weekly Epidemiological Record* 71: 289–291.

Joint WHO/UNICEF Statement. 1989. *Protecting, Promoting and Supporting Breastfeeding*. Geneva, Switzerland: World Health Organization.

Kingman, Sharon. 1993. Researchers confirm AIDS epidemic in Africa. *British Medical Journal* 306: 1564.

Kinoshita, K. S. Hino, et al. 1984. Demonstration of adult T-cell leukemia virus antigen in milk from three sero-positive mothers. *Gann* 75: 103–105.

Kumar, Rachana M., Sayenna A. Uduman and Ashok K. Khurranna. 1995. A prospective study of mother-to-infant HIV transmission in tribal women from India. *Journal of Acquired Immune Deficiency Syndromes* 9: 238–242.

Labbok, M., G. Grave, M. Forman. 1981. Summary of the workshop on the determinants of the choice and duration of infant feeding practices. National Institute of Child Health and Development, June 9–11.

Labbok, M., B. Klaus and D. Barker. 1983. Factors related to ovulation method efficiency in three programs: Bangladesh, Kenya and Korea. *Contraception* 37: 577–589.

Labbok, M. 1984. Contraception during lactation: Considerations in advising an individual or family planning program. *Population Forum*, First Issue.

_____. 1985. Contraception during lactation: Considerations in advising the individual or in formulating programme guidelines. In *Breast-feeding and Fertility*, eds. Malcolm Potts et al. Madison, Conn: Research Books, pp. 55–56.

Labbok, Miriam, and Katherine Krasovec. 1989. The role of U.S.-based organizations. *Institute for Reproductive Health Report* 5, June.

_____. 1990. Toward consistency in breastfeeding definitions. *Studies in Family Planning* 21: 226–230.

Labbok, M. 1991. Rejoinder to Trussell and Santow (in response to "Is the Bellagio Consensus Statement on the Use of Contraception Sound Public Health Policy?"). *Health Transition Review* 1: 111–114.

Labbok, M., et al. 1994. The lactational amenorrhea method: A postpartum introductory family planning method with policy and program implications. *Advances in Contraception* 10: 93–109.

Labbok, Miriam H. 1997a. Consultation on Infants and AIDS. Community Nutrition Institute, Washington, D.C., July 17.

Labbok, Miriam H., et al. 1997b. Multicenter study of the lactational amenorrhea method (LAM): I. Efficacy, duration, and implications for clinical application. *Contraception* 55: 327–336.

La Leche League International. 1997. *Role of Mother's Milk in HIV Transmission Remains Unclear*. Schaumburg, Illinois: La Leche League International.

Lallemant, Marc, et al. 1989. Mother-child transmission of HIV-1 and infant survival in Brazzaville, Congo. *AIDS* 3: 643–646.

Lallemant, M., et al. 1991. Assessing the risk for mother-infant HIV-1 transmission: A challenge in resource-poor countries. Presented at the Seventh International Conference on AIDS, Florence, Italy, June 16–21.

_____. 1994. Mother-to-child transmission of HIV-1 in Congo, Central Africa. *AIDS*. 8: 1451–1456.

Le Coeur, Sophie, and Marc Lallemant. 1996. Pediatric HIV/AIDS. In *Aids in the World II*, eds. Jonathan Mann and Daniel Tarantola. New York/Oxford: Oxford University Press, pp. 273–277.

Lepage, Philippe, et al. 1987. Postnatal transmission of HIV from mother to child. *Lancet* ii: 400.

Machekanyange, Zorodzai. 1997. Zimbabwe: Is breast milk still best? *Africa Information Afrique*. Harare, Zimbabwe, September 8.

Meier, Barry. 1997. In war against AIDS, battle over baby formula reignites. *New York Times*, June 8, pp. 1, 16.

Minkoff, H., D. Nanda, R. Menez and S. Fikrig. 1987. Pregnancies resulting in infants with acquired immunodeficiency syndrome or AIDS-related complex: Follow up of mothers, children and subsequent born siblings. *Obstetrics and Gynecology* 69: 285–287.

Mok, J. Q., et al. 1987. Infants born to HIV seropositive mothers: Preliminary findings from a multi-centre European study. *Lancet* I: 1164–1168.

Narayan, O., and L. C. Cork. 1985. Lentiviral diseases of sheep and goats: Chronic pneumonia leukoencephalomyelitis and arthritis. *Review of Infectious Diseases* 7: 89–98.

Nduati, Ruth. 1998. *HIV and Infant Feeding: A Review of HIV Transmission Through Breastfeeding.* UNICEF/UNAIDS/WHO.

Pan American Health Organization. 1990. Report of the International Conference on Maternal-Infant AIDS in the Americas. Washington, D.C.: PAHO, August.

Piot, Peter. 1997. Fighting AIDS together. In *The Progress of Nations 1997*. New York: UNICEF.

Pitts, M., and H. Jackson. 1993. Press coverage of AIDS in Zimbabwe. *AIDS Care* 5: 223–230.

Raphael, Dana. 1994. The politics of international health: Breastfeeding and HIV. In *Global AIDS Policy*, ed. Douglas A. Feldman. Westport, Conn.: Bergin and Garvey, pp. 129–141.

Rubini, N. P. M., et. al. 1996. HIV vertical transmission in Rio de Janeiro: Rate and risk factors. Presented at the Eleventh International Conference on AIDS, Vancouver, July 7–12. Abstract Tu.C.2570.

Saadeh, Randa J., Miriam H. Labbok, Kristin A. Cooney and Peggy Koniz-Booher, eds. 1993. *Breast-feeding: The Technical Basis for Action.* Geneva, Switzerland: World Health Organization.

Senturia, Y. D., A. E. Ades, C. S. Peckham and C. Giaquinto. 1987. Breastfeeding and HIV infection. *Lancet* 2: 400.

Shilts, Randy. 1987. *And the Band Played On.* New York: St. Martin's Press.

Simonon, Arlette, et al. 1994. An assessment of the timing of mother-to-child transmission of human immunodeficiency virus type 1 by means of polymerase chain reaction. *Journal of Acquired Immune Deficiency Syndromes* 7: 952–957.

Stamps, Timothy. 1997. Address to the World Health Assembly, Geneva, Switzerland, May.

*Status and Trends of the Global HIV/AIDS Pandemic, Official Satellite Symposium, July 5-6, 1996.* AIDSCAP, François-Xavier Bagnoud Center for Health and Human Rights of Harvard School of Public Health and UNAIDS.

Swazi babies in hospital with HIV virus. 1995. *Reuters News Service*, March 1.

Taha, Taha E., et al. 1995. The effect of human immunodeficiency virus infection on birthweight, infant and child mortality in urban Malawi. *International Journal of Epidemiology* 24(5): 1022–1029.

Teich, N., et al. 1984. Pathogenesis of retrovirus-induced disease. In *RNA Tumor Viruses*, eds. N. Teich, H. Varmus and J. Coffin. Cold Spring, New York: Cold Spring Harbor Laboratory, pp. 785–798.

Teply, L. J. 1979. Breastfeeding, milk and UNICEF. In *Breastfeeding and Food Policy in a Hungry World*, ed. Dana Raphael. New York: Academic Press, pp. 253–258.

Thiry, L., et al. 1985. Isolation of AIDS virus from cell-free breast milk of three healthy virus carriers. *Lancet* ii: 891–892.

Turmen, S. 1997. *HIV and Infant Feeding.* Draft Statement for the WHA 1997.

UNAIDS Joint United Nations Programme on HIV/AIDS. 1996. HIV and Infant Feeding: An Interim Statement. *Weekly Epidemiological Record* 71: 289–291.

_____. 1997a. *Breastfeeding and HIV/AIDS.* Geneva, Switzerland: UNAIDS.

_____. 1997b. *Report on the Global HIV/AIDS Epidemic.* Geneva, Switzerland: UNAIDS.

_____. 1998. International meeting calls for concerted action to prevent mother-to-child transmission of HIV. Press release, Geneva, Switzerland, March 24.

UNICEF. 1996a. *Promise and Progress: Achieving Goals for Children.* New York: UNICEF.

_____. 1996b. *Fifty Years for Children.* New York: UNICEF.

_____. 1998. *New HIV/AIDS Treatment Will Save Thousands of Children.* New York: UNICEF, March 26.

Van Esterik, Penny. 1989. *Beyond the Breast-Bottle Controversy.* New Brunswick, New Jersey: Rutgers University Press.

Waldholz, Michael. 1998. AZT price cut for Third World mothers-to-be. *Wall Street Journal*, March 5, p. B1.

Weinbreck, P., et al. 1988. Postnatal transmission of HIV infection. *Lancet* i: 482.

World Health Organization. 1987. Breast-feeding: Breast milk and human immunodeficiency virus (HIV). *Weekly Epidemiological Record* 33: 245–246.

World Health Organization Global Programme on AIDS. 1992. Consensus statement from the WHO/UNICEF Constitution on HIV transmission and breast feeding. *Weekly Epidemiological Record.* 67:177–184.

World Health Organization, UNAIDS and UNICEF. 1998. *Technical Consultation on HIV and Infant Feeding, Geneva, Switzerland, April 20–22.* Conclusions.

Ziegler, John B., David A. Cooper, Richard O. Johnson and Julian Gold. 1985. Postnatal transmission of AIDS-associated retrovirus from mother to infant. *Lancet* ii: 896–897.

# PART FOUR:

## Decisions About Infant Feeding

CHAPTER EIGHT

# The Fears
# Driving Women's
# Infant Feeding Decisions

There is an ominous quality to the early reports on women's fears about transmitting HIV in their breastmilk and their fears of stigmatization. This chapter outlines the early reports about the effect of women's beliefs concerning AIDS on their feeding practices and attitudes.

## Women Spontaneously Choose to Formula Feed

The phenomenon whereby HIV-negative and untested women avoid breastfeeding has been called the "spillover" effect. If health workers distribute formula or if they waiver in their support of breastfeeding, it can contribute to this effect in the future. But women have actually been "spilling over" into the non-breastfeeding group since the late 1980s, and it had nothing to do with formula distribution; there wasn't any. Nor did the abandonment of breastfeeding have anything to do with any policy recommendations on infant feeding; women were advised to keep breastfeeding. Rather, "spillover" happened spontaneously. Nicoll had predicted in 1990 that a switch to bottle-feeding would occur naturally as women became aware of the possibility of transmitting the virus in their milk.

Years ago, psychologists urged researchers to include components in their trials to assess women's well-being and decision-making capacities. Such appraisals, however, "have consistently been rejected in favour of the hard science of knowing numerical transmission rates — rather than knowing what this means for the women who might be passing the virus to their children" (Gorna 1996:245–246). Sherr (1998) also noted that psychological aspects of infant feeding have been omitted from research to date. She urged that future research encompass psychological data, including mothers' opinions.

Ten years after public health officials knew that a Zairian radio broadcast had caused women to abandon breastfeeding, research on mothers' reactions and on breastfeeding avoidance is still lacking. It remains to be seen how breastfeeding will be promoted among women who know that it can transmit the AIDS virus.

In most of the world, however, HIV/AIDS is still at low levels, and breastfeeding programs are not being impacted by AIDS-related fears. Women first have to hear that breastmilk can transmit HIV and feel that this may affect them. But contrary to popular belief, populations with very low levels of AIDS do not dismiss its threat as remote or irrelevant. Surveys done in 16 countries in Africa, Asia and South America found no support for the idea that people in low prevalence areas don't worry about AIDS (Cleland 1995:162). Thus even some women in low prevalence areas who hear that breastmilk can transmit AIDS may be susceptible to fears. Satellite television is speeding up the spread of information faster than radio.

In the future, it seems unlikely that the simple "breast is best" advice will suffice, even among uninfected women, especially if they fear that their male partners may infect them at any time. There are anecdotal reports from the United States of tested HIV-negative women insisting that they are avoiding breastfeeding because of AIDS— despite much counseling and reassurance about their seronegativity. Perhaps these women mistrust their male partners. Perhaps it is just an excuse not to breastfeed. Perhaps we do not understand breastfeeding avoidance as well as we must.

## Women Who Did or Did Not Know That Breastfeeding Transmits HIV

Despite some reports, most African women, even HIV-infected women, have continued to breastfeed. But women's reasons for doing so bear little resemblance to the reasons advanced by the breastfeeding promoters. The breastfeeding promoters cite reduced diarrhea (Bellamy 1998), reduced fertility (Short 1991), and the financial burden on nations that try to provide breastmilk substitutes (Berg 1997). The promoters also point to calculations that show that breastfeeding by HIV-infected women is safer under the worst conditions in resource-poor countries (Hu 1992, Del Fante 1993). The promoters also cite the need to protect breastfeeding efforts (Nicoll 1995, Kuhn and Stein 1997, UNAIDS 1997, Geloo 1998).

But the HIV-infected women who have continued to breastfeed have not done so for these reasons. Most HIV-infected women continued to breastfeed because they didn't know that they were infected, didn't know that breastmilk can transmit HIV, or didn't want their male partners to find out that they are HIV-positive. Many have continued to feed as they otherwise would have, in what amounts to partial prolonged breastfeeding.

Women in India in the mid–1990s knew almost nothing about HIV, never mind about *breastfeeding* and HIV (Kapila 1997). In many cultures women are not free to make informed decisions. If the mother-in-law or some other family member decrees breastfeeding, then breastfeeding it will be. The control of breastfeeding is a male prerogative in many societies (Maher 1995:11).

In Africa, where the virus has been known longest, being untested is not necessarily the same as being uninformed. Most urban-educated mothers in Rwanda associated breastfeeding with HIV transmission (O'Gara 1996). Women in Rwanda said that, even if health workers told women with AIDS to breastfeed, they would not do so. "I would probably kill myself and give the baby to my family to raise" (Wellstart 1994). When 680 breastfeeding women in Nigeria were interviewed, none said she would breastfeed if HIV-infected (Ighogboja 1995).

In rural Zimbabwe, two-thirds of the women knew that breastfeeding can transmit HIV, and many were bottle-feeding (Gregson 1998). In Soweto, South Africa, 97 percent of the HIV-positive mothers who did not breastfeed said that this was because they were worried about transmitting HIV to their babies (Urban 1997).

## Those Who Have Been Forced to Breastfeed Because of Cultural Norms

By the mid–1990s, more than 95 percent of HIV-infected women in Tanzania knew that breastfeeding can transmit HIV, "but because of cultural norms they were forced to keep on breast feeding their babies" (Mutembei 1997). The other major reason was poverty; HIV-infected women in Tanzania said that they breastfed because they could not afford formula.

In Cape Town, South Africa, 77 percent of HIV-positive women knew that breastfeeding can transmit HIV. Most actually believed, incorrectly, that all breastfed babies would become HIV-infected (Kuhn 1997). Nevertheless, 94 percent of HIV-positive women breastfed; 92 percent were motivated by fear of telling family members that they were HIV-positive.

Women have good cause to fear a diagnosis and disclosure of seropositivity. It is not uncommon for a man to abandon his wife when he learns that she is HIV-infected (Auer 1996). Danziger (1994) quoted a doctor in Zaire as saying, "If we tell the husband that his wife is HIV-positive, he'll blame it on her and leave her and the children."

Dr. Stefan Wiktor of the CDC–Côte d'Ivoire clinical trial, which is studying short-term AZT, noted that half of the women who tested positive did not inform their partners. Wiktor noted, "These women are almost entirely economically dependent on men, and we suspect they fear stigmatization and abandonment" (Feinman 1997).

In Brazil, HIV-infected mothers who breastfed were asked why they had done so. Sixty percent breastfed because they did not learn their HIV status before leaving the maternity hospital. Eighteen percent were never told that breastfeeding can transmit HIV. Twenty-two percent breastfed despite counseling either because they did not believe that breastfeeding can transmit HIV or because they could not afford formula (Tess 1997).

In a study of 70 HIV-positive women in Soweto, South Africa, HIV-positive women were told of the benefits and risks of breastfeeding, but they were allowed to make their own informed decisions. According to researchers Urban, Gray and Wagstaff (1997), of the 70 women, 35 breastfed. Those who breastfed were more likely to have received only one counseling session and may not have understood the risks. Some of these women said they breastfed because they could not afford formula.

Pediatrician Glenda Gray, who was one of the researchers in the work in Soweto, noted that some of the HIV-positive mothers felt compelled to hide their status from family members. So they made up excuses for bottle-feeding, often claiming they didn't have enough breastmilk for the baby. Gray described a mother who pretended to breastfeed in front of her family by latching the baby on, way off to the side of her breast. Then she secretly fed her baby formula.

Gray reported that at one time she herself was buying formula at the "state price," which is about one-third of the store price, and selling it to HIV-infected mothers at cost. Conceding that this put her in conflict with the WHO Code, Gray said, "I'm dying for someone to take me to court for it. ... What's more important? Upholding a breastfeeding code that is inflexible and allows children to die, or saving lives?" (Lerner 1998). After formula was supplied to HIV-positive mothers in Soweto, many more totally avoided breastfeeding their babies (Gray 1998).

## HIV-Infected Mothers, Breastfeeding and Fatalism

Another reason why HIV-infected women breastfeed is fatalism. Strebel (1996) listed fear, fatalism and denial of risk as the significant reasons why women do not protect themselves against sexual contact with HIV-infected men. Likewise, some women in Uganda expressed resignation about risks associated with breastfeeding while HIV-infected. They said that a mother "might as well breastfeed until they both die.... What else can she do?" (Nutrition Division 1994). Other women may just hope that their milk doesn't infect their babies. Ultimately, many mothers breastfeed because they believed it to be an intrinsic part of motherhood for them and not to breastfeed seems unthinkable.

## Our Analyses, Women's Perceptions

Analyses have shown that, under the very worst conditions (no clean water, no provision of safe replacement feeding), there are fewer overall deaths projected if HIV-infected women continue to breastfeed at least for a few months (Heymann 1990, Hu 1992, Del Fante 1993, Kahn 1997, Kuhn and Stein 1997). All analyses show that overall deaths are fewer if an entire population of untested women continues to breastfeed. But Carol Gilligan (1982) noted that women "de-emphasize logical rules imposed by social institutions, mostly run by men." Gilligan described the young woman's sense of morality, which is a relevant issue here. It is young women who give birth to most babies. According to Gilligan, young women see moral values in a personal, contextual view of life. They seek connectedness to others. When faced with conflict, they tend to want to change the rules to avoid conflict. Thus women may be willing to change the rule from "breastfeed" to a new rule: "Don't breastfeed if you think you might have the AIDS virus."

Breastfeeding pioneer Dr. Niles Newton used the phrase *aggressive protection* to refer to the way that mothers will safeguard their young (Newton 1955:99). Mothers have been observed to do incredible things to keep their children alive. It is not rational for starving people to give away their food, but starving mothers do it all the time; they give their food to their children. This is why more young children survive famines than might be rationally predicted. It is an act of unusual heroism for starving people to give away most of their food only when they are not mothers. Eritrean women in Sudanese refugee camps "unweaned" children who had already been weaned by putting them back to breast, thereby triggering the production of milk again (Almedom and de Waal 1990). This could hardly have been good for the severely malnourished women, but they did it to keep their children alive.

It may not be rational for women to have unprotected sex with men who may be HIV-infected, but some women have occasionally done so because it is the only feasible way to pay for food. When asked about prostitution, one woman replied, "HIV kills in three to ten years; hunger kills in three days. I have three children. Why should we starve if I can get money for immediate use?" (Paterson 1996:18)

Perhaps ever since the late 1980s, when it was first observed that some women were afraid to breastfeed, policy makers suspected that women would not want to breastfeed if they thought they might transmit a deadly virus to their children. Hence the silence on this issue. Perhaps, too, policy makers suspected that mothers would be unimpressed if they heard about the rational population-based analyses.

## Women Will Move Mountains to Have a Healthy Baby

Women at the 1998 International Conference on AIDS in Geneva expressed their feelings about breastfeeding by HIV-infected mothers. Mercy Maklamena, an HIV-positive woman from South Africa, addressed a plenary session and reminded participants that women will move mountains to have a healthy baby. She informed the audience that though her baby was put on AZT at birth, no one told her not to breastfeed. Her baby died of AIDS. She suggested that networks of PWAS (persons with AIDS) be trained to help women make fully informed decisions.

Lynde Francis (1998), who has been HIV-positive for 12 years and who works with the Centre for People Living with HIV in Harare, Zimbabwe, told participants at the Geneva Conference the story of her HIV-positive friend. The friend saw herself as having been forced to breastfeed and sees her child's death as being caused by breastfeeding. The woman had not been given any advice about breastfeeding through official channels, but learned about it by word of mouth. Because the baby appeared healthy for a while but later became symptomatic during continuing breastfeeding, the woman now says, "God saved my child. Now I, in my ignorance, have killed her." One could make the argument that the woman does not know for certain whether her child was infected by breastfeeding or during childbirth. But the woman perceives that she infected her child through breastfeeding, and it is women's perceptions — not rational arguments — that determine how they feed their babies, and what they say to other women.

Francis noted that women are not interested in mortality and morbidity calculations, and that *any* risk of HIV transmission is too much for a woman to take knowingly. She said she felt that women cannot be put on AZT and then breastfeed.

Other women attending the Geneva session organized by the International Community of Women Living with HIV/AIDS noted that women who learn of their seropositivity during their pregnancies often decide not to have more children. Thus the baby they carry — their only baby — is very precious.

At another session at the Geneva Conference, an African woman who did not give her name went to the microphone to urge representatives of the World

Health Organization to include in its HIV and infant feeding discussions women from resource-poor countries.

Rebecca Denison, an HIV-positive U.S. woman, expressed the feeling that women are seen as not being intelligent enough to make infant feeding decisions. Denison is associated with Women Organized to Respond to Life-threatening Diseases (WORLD).

At a 1996 conference in South Africa, an HIV-positive woman noted that her infant daughter had died two weeks earlier. The woman wondered aloud if her daughter would be alive if she had been bottle-fed: "If our babies could speak, they would say, 'We don't want our mother's milk, if it will infect us'" (Humphrey 1996).

It is not surprising that women who have watched children die from AIDS and children die from unsafe bottle-feeding or gruel-feeding may be less repulsed by the latter. Nicoll and colleagues (1995) commented, "Parents might prefer to risk their child's early death from diarrhoea rather than raise an HIV-1-infected child who will die following multiple dehabilitating illnesses."

Reid (1997:164) noted that, for HIV-positive women, two primary emotions dominate virtually every minute of the day: anger and guilt. Their anger is directed toward the person who infected them; their guilt is often self-directed "because they have so often infected one or more of their children."

## Excuses for Bottle-Feeding

Indian physician Damania, who presented a poster session at the 1998 Geneva Conference, said that he helps some HIV-positive women find excuses to explain why they're not breastfeeding. He, for instance, has the women tell their families that they cannot nurse because his medical orders forbid breastfeeding after a cesarean delivery. While it is their seropositivity (not cesarean delivery) that is the real reason for breastfeeding avoidance, Damania stated that he is pleased to allow women to use his medical orders as the reason they give to relatives for not breastfeeding. He has advised other HIV-positive women to cover themselves and their babies with blankets so that onlookers do not see them bottle-feeding.

## It Is Known — Make It Felt

At the beginning of their book *AIDS in the World II*, Mann and Tarantola quote lines from a play about an earlier plague. One character says that he will make their troubles known. Another character replies: "It is known. Everyone knows our trouble, that is why we are shunned. Make it felt."

For women who watch children die from AIDS, it is felt. But for others it may be merely known. Elizabeth Glaser's description of how she infected her daughter with her breastmilk makes her experience felt. Elizabeth was a U.S. woman who first became well known because she was married to an actor, Paul Michael Glaser. Elizabeth told her story to the U.S. national television audience during the 1992 Democratic National Convention and again in her book *In the Absence of Angels* (1991).

When Elizabeth gave birth to her daughter Ariel in August 1981, it was only two months after the CDC had first reported that a few gay men in Los Angeles had an unusual form of pneumonia, *Pneumocystis carinii*. Unfortunately Elizabeth needed blood transfusions after her cesarean delivery, and she was transfused with HIV-infected blood. She then passed the virus on to her daughter via breastfeeding.

Around the time of Ariel's fourth birthday, in 1985, Ari became very ill with diarrhea, experiencing both fatigue and great pain. Elizabeth noted that Ari woke up in the night screaming in pain because she had to go to the bathroom. Finally, after many painful illnesses and months of testing, physicians discovered what was wrong with Ariel. She had AIDS. In her book, *In the Absence of Angels*, Elizabeth described the situation in 1987:

> Ariel was in withering pain from her pancreatitis. As she became sicker, our relationship became more intense and unlike any I have ever had with another human being. She and I became one even more powerfully now. I was feeling every ounce of her pain, every grimace.... [As of 1988] Ariel still looked like a wisp of life. She could open her eyes and was able to communicate by blinking.... The pain was monumental for her at times. The screams would move in silent contractions across her face and her body. It was as bad to see them as it had been to hear them.

Ari died in 1988 and Elizabeth died in 1994.

Elizabeth's 1992 speech on U.S. television was criticized for not presenting balanced information on the benefits of breastfeeding and the dangers of breastmilk substitutes for babies in the developing world (O'Gara 1996). The implication seems to be that she might have followed up the description of her daughter's suffering with some words about the advantages of breastfeeding and the dangers of Third World bottle-feeding.

## The Concept of "Bad Milk"

The concept of bad breastmilk is much more generally accepted in non–Western cultures. Women living in societies that accept the general idea of bad milk may be quicker than some Westerners to believe that things make breastmilk harmful to the child.

It is extremely common for people in various cultures to consider the colostrum (first breastmilk) bad (Van Esterik 1988:197). While Westerners see colostrum as full of antibodies and nutrients and as a wonderful early laxative for the newborn, people in many cultures see colostrum as unhealthful. They therefore either throw it out or wait until their mature milk comes in (Castle 1988:104). Women in Uganda differ in their views of colostrum, but only one group believes that colostrum is good for babies. All others describe it as "dirty," "thick," "watery," "yellow," "unclean," "full of disease organisms," or "hot." Some believe colostrum can scald the baby's mouth or cause diarrhea. Most Ugandan women discard all or part of it (Nutrition Division 1994). Even mature breastmilk may be thought of as bad. When women believe any breastmilk is bad, they usually choose not to breastfeed, reasoning that bad milk makes children sick.

In *The Anthropology of Breastfeeding*, Maher (1995:166) points out that beliefs about poisonous breastmilk are legion and include most cultures where women are overworked and underfed and bear many children. Maher suggests that the beliefs are useful because they get other people to take care of breastfeeding women. By saying that milk becomes poisonous if mothers become overtired or overheated, people are saying that mothers need to be relieved of burdens such as working in the hot sun. Other women can and do step in to relieve breastfeeding mothers of burdens that might make their milk bad.

This insight unfortunately may not be useful in dealing with AIDS. The best way to prevent a breastfeeding mother from having virus-laden breastmilk is not to take her out of the hot sun; it's to stop a society from believing that sexual access to women's bodies is a male birthright and that multi-partner unprotected intercourse is acceptable. Changing such beliefs is clearly much more difficult than taking women out of hot fields where they spend ten hours a day. The distribution of female condoms and the development of vaginal microbicides may help as stopgap measures.

The extent to which traditional beliefs about bad milk meld with ideas about AIDS is intriguing. Sex, people think, can make women lactate bad milk. Since women don't breastfeed when they believe their milk is tainted, it follows that women should abide by rules about sexuality. In some cultures it is thought to be especially important that women avoid new sexual partners while breastfeeding.

In Guinea-Bissau there are women who believe they start out with bad milk. As a result, they either choose not to breastfeed or they wean early (Jakobsen 1996). Why is their milk bad? The women probably committed adultery at some point (Gunnlaugsson 1993). Some people in Uganda also believe that sexual activity will affect breastmilk, particularly when the woman has had sex with a man who is not the baby's father. Women in some districts in Uganda believe that milk becomes contaminated if it is in a breast that is ever sucked on by a man (Nutrition Division 1994).

Some Mende women of Sierra Leone believe that semen contaminates milk, so they wean their babies to tinned milk. When they talk about breast-feeding and weaning, they talk about sex (Bledsoe 1987).

In Malawi, breastmilk reflects the moral standing of the mother and father and their faithfulness to one another. If the father is unfaithful and then touches his child, it is believed the child will die from a nosebleed. If the mother has sex outside of marriage, her lover's sperm will contaminate her milk. Even sex within marriage should be had in moderation; children will be delayed in learning to sit up or walk if they drink breastmilk with too much sperm from the parents' having intercourse every day (Obermeyer and Castle 1997).

Bad breastmilk can also result from malnutrition, or the wrong types of foods, or general poor health on the part of the mother. AIDS, called the "slim" disease in Africa, would seem to hurt breastmilk. In Tunisia, women's milk becomes unhealthful if they get tired and hot (Creyghton 1992). In Lebanon, women's milk becomes harmful if they get tired and angry (Harfouche 1981). Women in Brazil say that they are so tired and weak that their "infants can suck and suck and all they will ever get is blood and pus" (Scheper-Hughes 1992:326). People in Haiti see body fluids as moral barometers. If a Haitian woman is believed to have bad blood, she is likewise believed to lactate spoiled milk (Farmer 1988). In prior centuries people paid a great deal of attention to the health of the wet nurse, lest she infect her charge.

So although the concept of bad breastmilk may be anathema to Westerners, many people believe in it, and they probably find it logical to believe that AIDS can make breastmilk bad. In 1998, the Internet provided a forum for ideas on bad milk. From Fiji (Speith 1998) came two questions: Is it still a good idea to use breastmilk as eye drops? and What about men who love to drink breastmilk? From India came a reply (Gilada 1998). Using infected breastmilk as a medicine would be relatively risky. Men who love to drink breastmilk should be prepared for the risk they take, especially if they have bleeding gums or ulcers in the mouth or intestines.

Given the fact that many African women know that breastfeeding can transmit HIV, and given the widespread belief in bad milk, it is not surprising that untested women have questioned the safety of their milk. It is tragic that they are abandoning breastfeeding, but it is not surprising. Even men are becoming leery of bad breastmilk.

The general AIDS educational messages may be adding to the dilemma about infant feeding. AIDS messages tell people not to take any chance on transmitting HIV. All men — not just tested, certifiably HIV-positive men — should wear condoms to avoid transmitting the virus in their semen. Suppose after being exposed to this AIDS education message that *any* man can transmit the virus in his semen a mother reasons that *any* woman can transmit it in her milk. Perhaps she then concludes that she can transmit it in *her* milk. Why should she still want to breastfeed?

One can argue that there is no harm in widespread condom use, but enormous harm in a widespread switch from breastfeeding to bottle-feeding. Arguments do not necessarily convince people. All the men who reject condoms seem to be showing by their behaviors that they see a harm in universal condom use (such as decreased sexual pleasure). Men avoid condoms, because men dislike condoms. But — and here is a sobering thought — many women like baby bottles. If women had disliked bottles the way men dislike condoms, the entire Nestlé boycott and the WHO Code would have been unnecessary.

## Rethinking Basic Ideas About Breastfeeding

Some women in Africa now seem to be abandoning breastfeeding because their maternal instincts, their traditional beliefs and their fear of AIDS tell them to do so. This suggests a need to reevaluate a basic hypothesis about breastfeeding. The prevailing hypothesis has been that Third World women fail to breastfeed exclusively because they are duped by formula company propaganda. They are seen as needing education and protection from industry and are presumed uneducated, irrational or selfish.

Breastfeeding anthropologist Vanessa Maher (1995) proposes an alternative hypothesis. Maher suggests that, far from naïve and dull-witted, these women are rational. Overworked, underfed, undersupported women are being shrewd, she argues, in trying to pass some of the burden of infant feeding onto others. Formula feeding makes inroads on male cash income rather than on women's bodily resources. Maher (1995:8) notes, "Women, in bottle-feeding, give up the impossible task of compensating with their own bodies for the shortcomings of a social and material environment which is hostile to women and children, and attempt to offload some of the burden of parenting and food production onto men."

A woman who is surviving by working eight to ten hours a day in a field or factory away from home is rational in not breastfeeding exclusively. Telling her about the benefits of exclusive breastfeeding or the dangers of bottle-feeding will not change her situation.

Maher notes too that many societies have the means to provide appropriate foods for older babies and toddlers, but they choose to rely on lengthy breastfeeding instead. While food scarcity is common among women and children, grown men are usually well nourished. Overburdened women, she feels, are rational in choosing bottle-feeding as a means of transferring to men "some of the cost of reproduction, which they have been bearing alone on an ever slimmer budget of food, cash and vitality" (1995:174). Malnutrition and overwork strain even lactational efficiency.

Carter (1995:126) also suggests that overworked women are not acting irrationally when they opt to administer breastmilk substitutes but choose them because they allow other people to feed the baby. She also notes from her research that "women do not want to be 'told' how to feed their children, valuing instead the ordinariness of the views of other women" (1995:187).

## Women's Concerns Not on the Agenda

In the pre–AIDS era, UNICEF had noted that breastfeeding can be painful, tiring, and inconvenient and that it puts a nutritional stress on the mother (Grant 1985:31). In 1985's *The State of the World's Children* report, UNICEF quoted Dr. Michael Latham's description of the heavy demands that breast-feeding makes on mothers in East Africa:

> The protein intake of pregnant and lactating mothers in Africa is extremely low.... Physicians often see the wreck of a woman follow-ing frequent pregnancies on an unsatisfactory diet. She is usually thin, miserable, anemic and often apathetic, with dry scaly skin, some-times rather lusterless hair, often with an ulcer that is reluctant to heal, and some mouth lesions. (Grant 1985:90)

Food supplement programs for mothers are often ineffective because mothers give away most of the donated food to their children. For example, a program in Colombia gave food supplements to mothers, who in turn gave most of the food to their children, taking in only 133 of the 856 calories given to them (Herrera 1980).

In the pre–AIDS era, then, overworked women's avoidance of breastfeed-ing was sensible. Likewise, in this era when women are learning that breast-milk can transmit the AIDS virus, eschewing breastfeeding is rational. How can one argue that a woman who believes her milk can infect her baby is irra-tional in avoiding breastfeeding? Consider that women's male partners some-times abandon them for other women if they test positive. Are women not rational in avoiding testing? Consider the significant risk that originally HIV-negative women run of infecting their babies following their own primary infection during breastfeeding. Are women not acting logically in shunning breastfeeding if they suspect that their male partners engage in risky behav-iors? Women's analyses of the best thing for their baby may not lead them to the same conclusions as computer-generated analyses of what is best for entire populations (Populations should accept testing and feed according to their tested HIV status.) But it is difficult to make a convincing case that women's analyses are unsound or that their fears are unfounded.

Feeding a child at one's breast is a deeply intimate act. Writer Adrienne Rich (1976:261–262) described one Hindu style of female infanticide: "Some-times opium was placed on the mother's nipple and the child was allowed to suckle herself to death." Rich notes that this seems to her to be "an atrocity which ranks high on the list of perverse crimes against women." Some women might find atrocious the idea of knowingly feeding their babies potentially infectious breastmilk. Readers who could imagine themselves HIV-infected through a needle stick might find appalling the idea that they would be asked to knowingly donate blood to a loved one.

# References

Almedom, Astier, and Alex de Waal. 1990. Constraints on weaning: Evidence from Ethiopia and the Sudan. *Journal of Biosocial Sciences* 15: 22.

Auer, Carrie. 1996. Women, children, and HIV/AIDS. In *Women's Experiences with HIV/AIDS*, eds. Lynellyn D. Long and E. Maxine Ankrah. New York: Columbia University Press, pp. 236–263.

Bellamy, Carol. 1998. *The State of the World's Children.* New York: UNICEF.

Berg, Alan. 1997. Breast still best. *World Bank Office Memorandum: New and Noteworthy in Nutrition* 30: 8.

Bledsoe, C. H. 1987. Side-stepping the postpartum sex taboo: Mende cultural perceptions of tinned milk in Sierra Leone. In *The Cultural Roots of African Fertility Regimes.* Proceedings of the IFE Conference, Nigeria, February 25–March 1.

Carter, Pam. 1995. *Feminism, Breasts and Breast-Feeding.* New York: St. Martin's Press.

Castle, Mary Ann, Beverly Winikoff, Moeljono Trastotenojo and Fatimah Muis. 1988. Infant feeding in Semarang, Indonesia. In *Feeding Infants in Four Societies*, eds. Beverly Winikoff, Mary Ann Castle and Virginia Hight Laukaran. New York: Greenwood Press, pp. 95–120.

Cleland, John, and Benoit Ferry. 1995. *Sexual Behavior and AIDS in the Resource-poor World.* London: Taylor & Francis, on behalf of the World Health Organization.

Coreil, Jeannine, et al. 1998. Cultural feasibility studies in preparation for clinical trials to reduce maternal-infant HIV transmission in Haiti. *AIDS Education and Prevention* 46: 46–62.

Creyghton, M. L. 1992. Breastfeeding and Baraka in Northern Tunisia. In *Anthropology of Breastfeeding*, ed. V. Mayer. Oxford: Berg Publishers, pp. 37–58.

Curtis, Hilary. 1997. *Breastfeeding and HIV?* Available from Gender-AIDS@bizet.inet.co.th; INTERNET. May 15.

Damania, Kaizad, et al. 1998. Three pronged strategy to prevent mother to child transmission. Presented at the Twelfth World AIDS Conference, Geneva, Switzerland, June 28–July 3. Abstract 23324.

Danziger, R. 1994. The social impact of HIV/AIDS in resource-poor countries. *Social Science and Medicine* 39: 905–917.

Del Fante, P., et al. 1993. HIV, breast-feeding & under-5 mortality: Modeling the impact of policy decisions for or against breast-feeding. *Journal of Tropical Medicine and Hygiene* 96: 203–211.

Farmer, Paul. 1988. Bad blood, spoiled milk: Bodily fluids as moral barometers in rural Haiti. *American Ethnologist* 51: 62–83.

Feinman, Jane. 1997. Tackling mother-to-child HIV in Côte d'Ivoire. *Lancet* 350: 1084.

Francis, Lynde. 1998. HIV-positive woman from Africa: A viewpoint on breast-feeding. In *Mother-to-Child HIV Transmission: Infant Feeding*. Presented at the Twelfth World AIDS Conference, Geneva, Switzerland, June 28–July 3.

Geloo, Zarina. 1998. HIV and Breastfeeding: Reigniting an old controversy. Women's Feature Service. *Women's International Net Magazine*. Available at http://www.geocities.com/wellesley/3321/win6d.htm; INTERNET.

Gilada, I. S. 1998. RE: Breast milk? Available from sea-AIDS @bizet.inet.co.th; INTERNET. February 20.

Gilligan, Carol. 1982. *In a Different Voice*. Cambridge, Massachusetts: Harvard University Press.

Glaser, Elizabeth, and Laura Palmer. 1991. *In the Absence of Angels*. New York: Berkley Books.

Gorna, Robin. 1996. *Vamps, Virgins and Victims: How Women Can Fight AIDS*. London: Cassell, Wellington House.

Grant, James P. 1985. *The State of the World's Children*. New York: UNICEF.

Gray, Glenda. 1998. Attitudes and behaviour of HIV-infected women on infant feeding. In *Mother-to-child HIV Transmission: Infant Feeding*. Presented at the Twelfth World AIDS Conference, Geneva, Switzerland, June 28-July 3.

Gregson, Simon, Tom Zhuwau, Roy Anderson and Stephen Chandiwana. 1998. Is there evidence for behavior change in response to AIDS in rural Zimbabwe? *Social Science and Medicine* 46: 321–330.

Greiner, Ted. 1997. The HIV threat to breastfeeding: Virus, fear and greed. Modified from a talk to the Bangladeshi Breastfeeding Foundation, August 29.

Gunnlaugsson, G., and J. Einarsdottir. 1993. Colostrum and ideas about bad milk: A case study from Guinea Bissau. *Social Science and Medicine* 36: 283–288.

Harfouche, J. K. 1981. The evil eye and infant health in Lebanon. In *The Evil Eye: A Folklore Casebook*, ed. A. Dundes. New York: Garland, pp. 86–106.

Herrera, M. G., J. O. Moore, B. DeParesdes and M. Wagner. 1980. Maternal weight/height and the effect of food supplementation during pregnancy and lactation. In *Maternal Nutrition During Pregnancy and Lactation: An Overview*, eds. H. Aebi and R. G. Whitehead. Bern: Hans Huber, pp. 213–227.

Heymann, Sally Jody. 1990. Modeling the impact of breast-feeding by HIV-infected women on child survival. *American Journal of Public Health* 80: 1305–1309.

Hu, D. J., et al. 1992. HIV infection and breast-feeding: Policy implications through a decision analysis model. *AIDS* 6: 1505–1513.

Humphrey, J. 1996. Report to Johns Hopkins School of Hygiene and Public Health about attendance at Workshop on Breast-feeding Choices for the HIV Seropositive Mother, Durban, South Africa, May 20–21.

Ighogboja, I. S., R. S. Olarewaju, C. U. Odumodu and H. O. Okuonghae. 1995.

Mothers' attitudes towards donated breastmilk, in Jos, Nigeria. *Journal of Human Lactation* 11: 93–96.

Interagency Group on Breastfeeding Monitoring. 1997. *Cracking the Code.* 1997. London: IGBM.

Jakobsen, Marianne S., Morton Sodemann, Kåre Molbak and Peter Aaby. 1996. Reason for termination of breastfeeding and the length of breastfeeding. *International Journal of Epidemiology* 25: 115–121.

Kapila, Bharucha, M. Ambekar and K. Khatri. 1997. Pretest counseling and HIV testing at antenatal clinic — Pune, India. Presented at the Conference on Global Strategies for the Prevention of HIV Transmission from Mothers to Infants, Washington, D.C., September 3–6.

Kahn, James. 1997. Infant feeding for HIV-infected mothers: Which strategies minimize mortality risk in different epidemiologic settings? Presented at the Conference on Global Strategies for the Prevention of HIV Transmission from Mothers to Infants, Washington, D.C., September 3–6.

Kuhn, Louise, et al. 1997. Child feeding practices and attitudes of HIV-positive mothers. Presented at the Conference on Global Strategies for the Prevention of HIV Transmission from Mothers to Infants, Washington D.C., September 3-6.

Kuhn, Louise, and Zena Stein. 1997. Infant survival, HIV infection, and feeding alternatives in less-developed countries. *American Journal of Public Health* 87: 926–931.

Lerner, Sharon. 1998. Striking a balance as AIDS enters the formula fray. *Ms.* VIII (5): 14–21, April.

Maher, Vanessa. 1995. *The Anthropology of Breast-Feeding: Natural Law or Social Constraint.* Oxford: Berg.

Maklamena, Mercy. 1998. Mother-to-child HIV transmission. Presented at the Twelfth World AIDS Conference, Geneva, Switzerland, June 28–July 3.

Mann, Jonathan, and Daniel Tarantola. 1996. Global Overview: The State of the Pandemic and its Impact. In *AIDS in the World II*, eds. Jonathan Mann and Daniel Tarantola, New York: Oxford University Press, pp. 5–40.

Mutembei, I. B. 1997. African cultural norms imposing breast-feeding to babies vis-à-vis HIV transmission during the breastfeeding period. Presented at the Conference on Affordable Options for the Prevention of Mother-to-child Transmission of HIV-1, Johannesburg, South Africa, November 19–20.

Newton, Niles. 1955. *Maternal Emotions.* New York: Paul B. Hoebner.

Nicoll, A., J. Z. J. Killewo and C. Mgone. 1990. HIV and infant feeding practices: Epidemiological implications for sub–Saharan African countries. AIDS 4: 661–665.

Nicoll, Angus, et al. 1995. Infant feeding policy and practice in the presence of HIV-1 infection. *AIDS* 9: 107–119.

Nutrition Division of the Uganda Ministry of Health, Child Health and Development Center of Makerere University and Wellstart International. 1994. *Breastfeeding in Uganda: Beliefs and Practices.* Washington, D.C.: USAID.

Obermeyer, C. M., and S. Castle. 1997. Back to nature? Historical and cross-cultural perspectives on barriers to optimal breastfeeding. *Medical Anthropology* 17: 39–63.

O'Gara, Chloe, and Anna C. Martin. 1996. HIV and breast-feeding: Informed choice in the face of medical ambiguity. In *Women's Experiences with HIV/AIDS*, eds. Lynellyn D. Long and E. Maxine Ankrah. New York: Columbia University Press, pp. 220–235.

Opperman, Edith. 1997. To breast-feed or not to breast-feed: That is the question in Zimbabwe. Presented at the Conference on Global Strategies for the Prevention of HIV Transmission from Mothers to Infants, Washington, D.C., September 3–6.

Paterson, Gillian. 1996. *Women in the Time of AIDS*. Maryknoll, New York: Orbis Books.

Reid, Elizabeth. 1997. Placing women at the center of analysis. In *AIDS in Africa and the Caribbean*, eds. George C. Bond, John Kreniske, Ida Susser and Joan Vincent. Boulder, Colorado: Westview Press, pp. 159–164.

Rich, Adrienne. 1976. *Of Woman Born*. New York: Norton.

Scheper-Hughes, N. 1992. *Death Without Weeping: The Violence of Everyday Life in Brazil*. Berkeley: University of California Press.

Sherr, Lorraine. 1998. Psychosocial aspects of breastfeeding. In *Mother-to-Child HIV Transmission: Infant Feeding*. Presented at the Twelfth International Conference on AIDS, Geneva, Switzerland, June 28–July 3.

Short, Roger. 1991. Report at a UN Administrative Committee on Coordination Subcommittee on Nutrition. Reported in *New & Noteworthy* (no. 15), ed. Alan Berg, November 13.

Speith, Jovesa. 1998. Breast milk? Available from sea-AIDS @bizet.inet.co.th; INTERNET. February 17.

Strebel, Anna. 1996. Prevention implications of AIDS discourses among South African women. *AIDS Education and Prevention* 8: 352–374.

Tess B. H., L. C. Rodrigues, M.-L. Newell and D. T. Dunn. 1997. Risk factors for mother-to-infant transmission of HIV-1 in São Paulo State, Brazil. Presented at the Fourth Conference on Retroviruses and Opportunistic Infections, Washington, D.C., January 22–27. Abstract 308.

UNAIDS. 1997. *HIV and Infant Feeding*. A Policy Statement. Geneva, Switzerland: UNAIDS.

Urban, Mike. 1997. Attitudes and practices of infant feeding in HIV-1 infected women in Soweto. Presented at the Conference on Affordable Options for the Prevention of Mother-to-Child Transmission of HIV-1, Johannesburg, South Africa, November 19–20.

Van Esterik, Penny. 1989. *Beyond the Breast-Bottle Controversy*. New Brunswick, New Jersey: Rutgers University Press.

Wellstart. 1994. *Qualitative Research on Breastfeeding in Kibungo and Gitarama Provinces*. Rwanda Ministry of Health.

Wiktor, Stefan Z. 1997. Trial in Côte d'Ivoire. Presented at the Tenth Conference on HIV and STDs in Africa, Abidjan, Côte d'Ivoire, December 7–11.

CHAPTER NINE

# Infant Feeding Alternatives For HIV-Infected Women

This chapter explores the alternatives to breastfeeding that have been suggested as ways to decrease mortality among babies of HIV-infected women. These are

- feeding generic formula
- feeding regular commercial formula
- feeding homemade "formulas" or animal milks and/or semisolid foods
- brief breastfeeding followed by rapid and complete cessation of breastfeeding
- wet-nursing
- use of antiretroviral drugs to treat breastfeeding mothers or babies
- feeding mother's own expressed and heat-treated breastmilk
- feeding heat-treated breastmilk from donors.

Women should be allowed to choose how they feed their babies but obviously can choose only from alternatives that are available and affordable to them. It should be noted that one alternative is already immediately available to all HIV-infected women, including women who live under the most difficult conditions: They can stop breastfeeding after the early months. But even this requires testing and counseling programs.

Those who hold the reins of power — governments and international health agencies — will decide whether, when and how to train health workers and whether to support other alternatives to breastfeeding. They are likely to make decisions based on affordability, feasibility and the desire to protect breastfeeding among uninfected women.

Women, on the other hand, will be guided by other concerns, such as the fear of infecting their babies, or their need to breastfeed to conceal seropositivity. Women may consider the relative stigmatization of various alternatives as important as policy makers consider affordability and the protection of breastfeeding. Nursing for three months and then stopping would be easier to explain away than cup-feeding a special generic formula that is provided only for tested, HIV-positive women. Breastfeeding while mother or baby takes AZT would be easier to explain away than hand expressing and heat-treating one's own breastmilk.

As more research results become available, recommendations that appear sound in 1999 may be modified. It is not yet known whether brief breast-feeding will offer good mortality protection or whether using AZT during breastfeeding will turn out to be feasible and effective.

## Different Points of View

We rank alternatives to breastfeeding through the lenses of our own cultures. Not only do women's perspectives differ from that of policy makers, the perspectives of some Westerners differ from one another. Researchers and breastfeeding advocates, for example, express different views about the appropriateness of various alternatives to breastfeeding.

Scientists have calculated that formula feeding is a very cost-effective way to prevent cases of HIV infection among people of all ages. World Bank's Nicholas Prescott, his colleagues from Thailand and the World Health Organization showed that, of all HIV preventive interventions, providing perinatal AZT and formula was by far the most cost-effective. It was much more cost effective than providing drug therapy for adults (Prescott 1996).

Lallemant and colleagues (1996) showed that, in developing countries, providing short-term AZT and bottle-feeding was cost-effective and compared favorably with most child survival interventions such as the prevention of diarrheal death. The World Health Organization had calculated that, with mixed-feeding, each diarrheal death averted had a price tag in the range of U.S.$1188-$4000 (Saadeh 1993:41).

Mansergh and colleagues from the CDC concluded that a national AZT program, in a setting with 12.5 percent seroprevalence, would be cost-effective at U.S.$1115 per infant HIV infection prevented (Mansergh 1996). With a 12.5 percent seroprevalence, then, preventing child deaths from AIDS is more cost effective than preventing deaths from diarrheal disease.

Söderlund and colleagues in Soweto, South Africa, noted that 44–94 percent of the cost of preventing mother-to-child infections rests with the screening costs. Combining formula feeding with perinatal interventions might therefore be highly cost effective, since the screening expense is incurred only once (Söderlund 1998).

Western breastfeeding advocates, on the other hand, emphasize alternatives that do not involve formula. They recommend as first consideration heat-treated mothers' milk, screened wet nurses and banked human milk (NABA 1997, La Leche League 1997). But a discussion paper from WABA, a breastfeeding advocacy group, pointed out the following: "The removal of breastmilk from the body except by a baby is a very recent and unnatural act." The paper also notes that since women rarely express breastmilk to save for later feedings, they are more likely to think that there is something wrong with breastmilk that has been expressed. The WABA paper notes the following about hand or pump expression: "No one likes it. It hurts, it's messy and it is not effective and there is no pleasure associated with it" (World Alliance for Breastfeeding Action, undated).

## Generic Formula

In 1998 UNICEF announced that it will begin some small projects to distribute generic formula for the babies of HIV-positive women in some resource-poor countries, including Botswana, Côte d'Ivoire, Rwanda, Uganda, Zambia, Cambodia and Vietnam. Six-month supplies of the formula "will be provided to tested women with HIV who make an informed choice to formula feed." It will be distributed at reduced cost through existing community-based institutions with careful control, targeting and monitoring (UNICEF 1998). Families will be counseled to be aware that formula can be fed by cup rather than by bottle. The WHO Technical Consultation (1998) recommended that generic formula be available only by prescription.

Mothers may make errors in formula preparation (Ho 1985), but they can with minimal instruction be taught how to prepare it correctly. Nduati (1998) noted that one of the major limitations of mathematical models supporting the promotion of breastfeeding is that "many of these models fail to consider that breast-milk substitutes can be used safely even in resource-poor setting if the women are well counseled thus reducing risks associated with diarrheal morbidity."

## Commercial Formula

Regular commercial formula is the obvious alternative for babies of HIV-positive women in industrialized nations, but for mothers in resource-poor countries, it is often too expensive. To those who can afford it, however, commercial formula may offer the advantage of being less stigmatizing than the special formula distributed only to tested HIV-positive mothers. Any woman using commercial formula would, of course have to admit that she is HIV-infected or come up with an excuse for not breastfeeding at all.

The WHO Technical Consultation (1998) noted that women have to know and accept their HIV status to make fully informed infant-feeding decisions. This statement is accurate, but not useful to women who cannot or will not be tested and who therefore will not be eligible for the affordable generic formula distributed by UNICEF and WHO. Untested women who avoid breastfeeding out of fear are likely to feed their babies whatever they can afford. It seems likely therefore that, in the immediate future, there will be more HIV-infected women feeding their babies overdiluted commercial formula than women who live in an area where the generic formula will be available and who will choose to know and accept their HIV status. Health workers may be trained to promote breastfeeding (and acceptance of seropositivity) for untested women, over bottle-feeding (and denial), but this does not mean that women will "comply."

## Homemade Formulas, Animal Milks and Semisolid Foods

In cultures where cattle, goats, buffaloes and camels are available, people have long used animal milk. Some African women attending the Twelfth World AIDS Conference stated their preference for using goat's milk — "not Nestlé." Noting the high number of goats in Africa and the many cows in the various regions, they proposed teaching women how to modify animal milks for their babies. Goat milk, deficient in folic acid and other nutrients, requires fortifying additives. According to the 1998 Guide for Health Care Managers and Supervisors, to modify milk from goats, cows or camels, one would dilute 100 milliliters of milk with 50 milliliters of boiled water and 10 grams (2 teaspoons) of sugar (UNICEF/UNAIDS/WHO 1998). This guide has other instructions for modifying animal milks, allowing health workers to teach women safe techniques for proper dilution, boiling water and adding other nutrients.

It has also been suggested that local communities might prepare homemade formulas out of local ingredients that are not milks. Soy, for instance, has become more common as a base for infant formulas in industrialized countries. Those pondering the use of soy may want to consider the various health problems associated with feeding the legume to infants, including problems with bowel mucosa (Ingkaran 1988), potential aluminum toxicity (Hawkins 1994), problems with absorption of minerals (Lonnerdal 1989), and the potentially adverse effects of soy plant estrogens. These expose infants to 6–11 times the level of plant estrogens known to have hormonal effects in adults (Clarkson 1995, Setchell 1997, Irvine 1995, 1998). Soy formulas may also interfere with immunization processes, as was noted with a rotavirus vaccine (Zoppi 1989) and with vaccines against polio, diphtheria, pertussis and tetanus vaccines (Zoppi 1983).

## Cup-Feeding

If mothers use cups to feed their babies formula or animal milks, they subsequently avoid the use of bottles, which tend to be more difficult to clean and thus may harbor bacteria. Rubber nipples (teats) tend to invite unhealthy bacteria, especially under the conditions of limited access to clean water and facilities that make hygiene inconvenient. A small feeding cup, powdered milk and soap constituted a home-feeding kit used by Mulago Hospital in Kampala, Uganda, in the 1960s. The feeding cup was made to be similar to the outer leaf of a banana flower, which was described as the traditional instrument used for feeding non-breastfed infants. The home-feeding kit was issued to be brought back weekly (Welbourn and De Beer 1964).

It is clear that a baby can be fed with a little cup that is held at the lower lip (Lang 1994). Mothers in the Nairobi randomized trial of breast versus formula feeding teach one another how to cup-feed, although bottles are sometimes used away from home (John, personal communication).

What is less clear is whether most mothers will want to use cups rather than bottles. People have talked for years about babies having "sucking needs," although there is no evidence one way or the other about their existence (Fisher 1996). But mothers may be guided less by science than by their own observations. Since bottle-feeding seems pleasurable to babies, and since mothers can cuddle their babies as they give them bottles, bottle-feeding may seem most like the breastfeeding that it is replacing. Bottle-feeding also allows older babies to hold their own bottles. Van Esterik (1989:175) noted that programs aimed at decreasing the use of bottles first need to understand what problems baby bottles solve for women.

The recommendation for cup-feeding is listed under the category of health care practices that can help to prevent spillover of untested women deciding not to breastfeed. Cup-feeding thus is considered protective of breastfeeding practices. Guidelines that call for health care professionals to ensure that mothers are taught to use cups to feed their infants, also state that no bottles should be given out (UNICEF/UNAIDS/WHO 1998b).

If other mothers in the community see cup-feeding as uninviting, it follows that they will be less likely to cup-feed. The cup-feeding of newborn babies is an uncommon sight in all cultures, but if it came to be known as the way HIV-infected mothers feed their babies, the stigmatization would make it even less appealing. HIV-infected women who are trying not to call attention to their seropositivity will probably find it easier to explain away bottle-feeding. Programs have taught women how to bottle-feed safely in Durban (Bobat 1997) and Soweto (Urban 1997), South Africa; in Yemen (Greiner 1997) and in Brazil (Rubini 1994).

## Early Cessation of Breastfeeding

Perhaps the major advantage of brief breastfeeding is that it is an immediately available option, even in the poorest villages of the most resource-limited countries. Where clean water is lacking and families have neither animals to milk nor money to buy formula or canned milk, brief breastfeeding appears to be a sensible alternative. Additionally, it has the advantage of being relatively non-stigmatizing.

While the risk of HIV infection through breastfeeding remains fairly constant, the risks associated with not breastfeeding decrease significantly after the early months. Slightly older infants can be weaned to local milks or semi-solid foods more easily than newborns.

Studies using PCRs show that some babies of HIV-infected mothers remain uninfected until they are 6 months old (Bertolli 1996, Ekpini 1997). In December 1997, Wiktor suggested that mothers in Côte d'Ivoire might be wise to cease breastfeeding at three months (Bunce 1997). Becquart (1998) and colleagues reported that six months of breastfeeding by mothers in the Central African Republic resulted in 52 percent of babies being HIV-infected. They suggested either three months of breastfeeding or none.

Mothers who stop breastfeeding early will, with the provision of some appropriate weaning foods and a little instruction, maximize nutrition and prevent "weanling diarrhea." It is the months after weaning that make up a critical time for children, including older babies or toddlers. Gordon (1963) noted that weanling diarrhea among children in the Punjab was a risk after weaning "irrespective of the particular age when that took place." Arguing that the quality of the weanling diet was very important, he noted the synergy between malnutrition and infection. Although diarrhea did occur shortly after weaning, deaths from diarrhea tended to happen later, as children's nutritional state and resistance to infection progressively deteriorated. This suggests that infected (and noninfected) women would benefit from ongoing help with selecting and preparing appropriate weaning foods. Since abrupt cessation of breastfeeding is not a common cultural practice, women will also benefit from practical advice, such as dealing with an unhappy infant and turning one's back on a cosleeping baby who can easily self-attach to the breast of a sleeping mother.

## Wet-Nursing

Wet-nursing, said to be the second oldest profession for women, is an accepted practice in many cultures where traditional guidelines exist, and it even affects other aspects of society. For example, according to Moslem tradition, two children nursed by the same wet nurse are considered milk siblings and therefore should not marry. People's feelings about wet-nursing vary. Women in one region of Mexico thought that wet-nursing was acceptable if needed, while those in another region, fearing that babies might become too attached to the wet nurse, were opposed to the practice (Perez-Gil 1996).

It has long been common for babies whose mothers died to be wet-nursed by their guardians. There have even been cases in which a non-lactating grandmother who, upon putting the orphaned grandchild to breast for comfort, began to lactate. It is now believed the grandmother in traditional cultures lactated for most of her adult life.

In HIV endemic areas today, grandmothers, sisters and aunts are taking in orphaned children. Some are likely putting babies to breast. Since there is no guarantee, however, that the wet nurse is uninfected, some health care professionals recommend "screened" wet nurses (La Leche 1997, NABA 1997). But screening is feasible only under circumstances in which HIV testing is available and desired. The UNICEF/UNAIDS/WHO (1998a) guidelines say that wet nurses should "be able to practice safe sex to remain HIV-negative while breast-feeding the infant."

Colebunders (1988) reported the first case of wet nurse–transmitted HIV. A woman in Zaire wet-nursed her nephew after her sister died during a cesarean delivery. (The dead woman had previously been in good general health, and although she had never been tested for HIV, her husband was HIV-negative.) The aunt breastfed the child for 12 months and died of AIDS when he was 17 months old. The child had symptoms of AIDS by the age of 11 months.

Wet-nursing not only poses a risk of woman-to-child HIV transmission, but also invites child-to-woman HIV transmission. Women who are contemplating wet-nursing the orphaned children of dead or dying HIV-infected mothers therefore need to be informed that they put themselves at risk.

One Russian report, in documenting the spread of HIV in a Soviet hospital, suggests that the risk to the wet nurse may be significant. A man apparently contracted HIV-1 when he was in West Africa. The virus was later identified as HIV-1, subtype G, linked to isolates common to Gabon, West Africa (Bobkov 1993, 1994). The man then infected his wife, who in turn passed the virus on to their unborn child (Fein 1989). At least one nurse reused a syringe for the infected infant and 27 other previously uninfected infants (Remnick 1989). (Some large Soviet hospitals used only one syringe per day.) The infected infants were then nursed at the breasts of previously uninfected mothers.

The first report (Belitsky 1989) of infant-to-mother transmission was initially met with skepticism. Testing conducted on one of the infant-mother pairs, however, indicated that the woman had indeed been infected by the child. Researchers investigated sequence variation of HIV-1 env gene encoding the V3 loop. They found that the V3 sequence clustered together in the analysis. All the HIV-1 infections in this cluster were subtype G, which suggests that all came from the original source (West Africa). Bobkov (1994) was unequivocal: "All individuals in this cohort were infected from a single viral source."

Pokrovsky (1991) estimated that 17 mothers became HIV-1-infected through cracks in their nipples while breastfeeding babies who were first infected via reused syringes. Bleeding gums in the infants and cracked nipples in the mothers may have facilitated transmission. Tiny cracks in nipples are common. Ziemer (1995) in the United States used magnified images of the nipples of 50 new mothers and found tiny fissures in the nipples of 76 percent of newly breastfeeding women. Women's subjective ratings of nipple soreness did not correlate with the presence of tiny nipple fissures.

Wet nurses, even if experienced breastfeeders, may develop nipple fissures. Traditional wet nurses often developed sore nipples when they took on a new baby, despite being expected to have toughened nipples. Even women who were nursing their own children when they began nursing others tended to experience nipple soreness. The new babies' more frequent and more intense nursing is thought to be the cause of the nipple soreness (Raphael 1973). It is a myth that only "modern" women (especially fair-skinned Caucasians) get sore nipples. Women in many cultures, whether nursing their own infants or those of others, experience sore and cracked nipples. Fildes (1986:140) described the beliefs that people in previous centuries had about nipple problems:

> Various reasons were given for the apparent high incidence of sore nipples, the main one being that hungry children, frustrated by getting insufficient milk, or not getting it easily, were liable to bite and "mump" the nipple. Whether or not the child had teeth, this led to sores which eventually could develop into ulcers.... Infants who suffered from conditions such as thrush ... were said to cause sore nipples in their nurses.

Oral thrush, or candida, is now known to cause sore nipples (Hoover 1997). Additionally, nipple fissures complicated by thrush may be very slow to heal. An orphaned baby infected before or during birth has a significant chance of developing candidiasis. In fact, in a study conducted in Uganda, 65 percent of 85 HIV-1-infected infants had candidiasis (Davachi 1994). In the United States, Kline (1996) found that most HIV-infected children in Texas had oral candida.

Since almost all children of HIV-infected mothers have unknown HIV status, adopting women should be informed of the risk they take if they decide to wet-nurse.

Another concern is that in some areas, it is common for women to casually offer the breast to any other woman's crying baby. The baby of an uninfected mother who is put to breast by several other women in the village is obviously at increased risk of infection in high prevalence areas. This point could be made to health workers.

## AZT Drug Therapy During Breastfeeding

Researchers have yet to determine whether treating breastfeeding mothers or babies with antiretroviral drugs such as AZT reduces the risk of transmission through breastfeeding, or even whether it is a feasible option. The rationale for treating breastfeeding mothers with the drugs is supported by research showing that AZT is excreted into breastmilk in levels that may be high enough to diminish its viral load (Ruff 1994). Whether the viral load will be reduced enough to make milk noninfectious over months of breastfeeding is not yet known. How well viral loads in blood correlate with viral loads in milk is also unclear.

On a theoretical level, it might be more logical to treat the mother, not the baby, with antiretroviral drugs during breastfeeding. Fiscus (1997) observed that treating mothers with AZT had been more effective in preventing mother-to-child HIV transmission than treating babies. She concluded this after looking back at mother-baby pairs who happened to have had various types of drug therapy. The retrospective study made use of records of HIV-infected mothers who gave birth to babies in North Carolina (USA) between 1993 and 1996.

But if mothers were treated with antiretroviral drugs for as long as breastfeeding typically lasts (one to two years), with the drug then withdrawn because of a lack of funding, virus rebound might result. Ethical concerns should require that a woman be considered for her own sake, not as a fetus-carrier or baby-feeder. A woman's own HIV disease might be negatively impacted by a breastmilk-focused drug therapy routine if she were disallowed to continue treatment.

Another concern is compliance patterns. Women would need to take the drugs at regular intervals. Also, if they are told to breastfeed for three months only while on AZT, it would be important for them to stop breastfeeding completely, lest they continue to breastfeed during a time when viral loads may possibly rebound following drug withdrawal.

Another option is to give an antiretroviral drug to breastfeeding babies to protect them from becoming HIV-infected as they ingest virus-laden breastmilk. Babies, if they remain uninfected, would need the drug only during the months of breastfeeding. Mothers would need to administer AZT syrup on a set schedule. Potential problems during treatment are side effects in the babies or missed dosages.

Researchers would need to follow children long-term to document whether there are any ill effects. Chemotherapeutic agents such as AZT appear to be remarkably safe, but they are given to newborn babies with caution and monitoring. Duration of safe breastfeeding would need to be determined, as would the cost of the antiretrorviral drug. None of the 1998 statements from the international health agencies recommends breastfeeding while mother or baby take AZT.

## Heat-Treating Mother's Milk

Eglin and Wilkinson (1987) reported that pasteurization inactivated HIV. They used two different commercial human milk pasteurizers to treat breast-milk, from uninfected donors, which had been spiked with tissue culture fluid containing HIV-infected cells. Orloff (1993) also showed that HIV is destroyed by pasteurization at 62.5° C as well as heat treatment at 56° C. But because some viruses such as CMV are not routinely destroyed at temperatures of 56° C, it is avised that milk be pasteurized at 62.5° C (Arnold 1996). The recommendation of UNICEF is that, if breastmilk is pasteurized, it should be done at 62.5° C for 30 minutes (Bellamy 1998).

Unfortunately pasteurization at 62.5° C results in a significant loss of some living protective components in breastmilk. While 100 percent of lysozyme is retained, only 22 percent of lactoferrin and 51 percent of IgA remain. Pasteurization at 62.5° C destroys the IgM and milk cells that might otherwise have protected babies against bacteria and viruses (Lawrence 1989:477–478). Narayanan (1984) reported that heating breastmilk to 62.5° C for 30 minutes significantly reduced its protective effect with babies in India.

If HIV-infected women hand express their breastmilk, heat-treat it, let it cool and then cup or bottle-feed it to the babies, they do not need breastmilk substitutes. This spares babies from being exposed to cow milk or other potential allergenic substances. But this plan is probably more difficult to keep secret than any other alternative to breastfeeding.

Many of the same requirements for minimizing the risk of bottle-feeding would also apply to expressed human milk. Women would need fuel for heat treatment, suitable containers with lids for heating their milk, and water and facilities for cleaning containers. They would need information on gauging time and temperature, and on preventing bacterial growth. Mothers usually feed according to infants' signals; this would not fit well with the need to allow time for the milk to cool to body temperature.

A suggestion was made in the United States that HIV-infected women might get help with the logistical problems of heat-treating their breastmilk at home by asking a milk bank to pasteurize it. But Lois Arnold, executive director of the Human Milk Banking Association of North America, commented,

> People not in the field of milk banking are being highly presumptuous and naïve to assume that milk banks would ever knowingly take milk that had the potential to be contaminated with HIV....The idea that milk banks, who are struggling financially anyway, would undertake to do the labor intensive, dangerous and liability-laden task of pasteurizing an HIV-positive mother's milk at NO COST is ludicrous and not based in reality. (Arnold 1998)

But there are more significant concerns about the feeding of heat-treated breastmilk. First, most women don't like expressing milk, and most cultures find it strange. Secondly, most women have a great deal of difficulty in keeping up their milk supply in the total absence of suckling. There are success stories of extremely dedicated mothers keeping up their milk supply for babies who were very premature or who had a condition such as an extensive cleft palate that made sucking impossible, but these women are the exception. Most mothers who try to collect milk long-term fail to do so. Even working mothers who get some nipple stimulation often find it challenging to keep up their milk stores.

Women in the U.S. who were using breast pumps to collect milk for their hospitalized premature infants were producing only 93 ml/day despite receiving counseling and despite increasing the number of times they expressed their milk (Ehrenkranz and Ackerman 1986). After taking the drug metoclopramide, the women's milk production increased to 197 ml/day, although the beneficial effect on milk volume is temporary, and even this higher amount is a very low milk supply. It was estimated that well-nourished women produce 600 milliliters in the first month and 800–1100 milliliters in the sixth month (Dewey and Lonnerdal 1983). A backup plan would be needed should mothers not collect enough breastmilk.

Local health workers who participated in a workshop in South Africa rejected as unfeasible the idea of asking women to express and heat-treat their breastmilk.

Plans for hand expressing breastmilk would be workable only in cultures where women are comfortable with the practice. Women in Rwanda had "strong negative feelings about expressing breastmilk" (Wellstart 1994). Women in Uganda also had especially negative feelings about expression of breastmilk: "Women expressed amazement, disbelief, amusement, or almost horror at the idea of expressing breastmilk to feed to a baby. 'It is never done.' One mother said: 'only cows are expressed' and another, 'if you are found doing it people will think you are a witch'" (Nutrition Division 1994). A mother-in-law was seen rushing out of a hospital room screaming that her daughter-in-law was a witch because she had expressed breastmilk into a cup. The cup, it was believed, needed to be destroyed because an adult who touched it, especially an in-law, would die.

## Use of Donor Breastmilk

Heat-treated donor breastmilk is a safe, nonallergenic food. Major barriers are cost, availability and feasibility. Nduati (1994), who had reported the case of a baby in Nairobi who apparently became HIV-infected by being fed raw breastmilk recommended heat treatment. Milk banks in North America dispense only heat-treated donor milk. They also screen donors by blood test and by history to ensure protection. The milk bank in Leipzig, Germany, however, supplies raw breastmilk, although it screens its donors every two months (Springer 1997).

Reported experiences in using donor breastmilk in the case of HIV infection are limited. In the United States, public funds were used to buy banked donor milk for one HIV-positive baby whose mother had died of AIDS and whose grandmother was caring for him. The average U.S. price, the so-called processing fee, is $2.50/ounce, although this falls far short of covering the true cost of producing an ounce of safe donor milk (Arnold 1997).

The Connecticut WIC program bought donor milk because the baby in question was HIV-positive, and it was hoped that the heat-treated breastmilk would help his immune function. But the grandmother-caregiver decided that she did not want to continue with the inconvenience of defrosting donor breastmilk, and she put the baby on formula (Arnold, personal communication).

In industrialized countries with widespread use of antiretroviral drugs for pregnant women, the overwhelming majority of babies born to treated HIV-positive mothers would be HIV-negative and would not be expected to have immune deficiency. Whether public funding would cover donor milk at more than U.S.$1000 per month per baby is questionable. In resource-poor countries the challenge would be the logistics of finding enough donors, heat-treating their milk, freezing or chilling it and then dispensing it to babies wherever they lived.

## The Informed Choice of Women

HIV-positive women are to be supported in whatever informed feeding choice they make. HIV-positive women will be switching from whatever feeding method they would have used had they been HIV-negative. Most women practice mixed breast and bottle-feeding. So, if they are HIV-positive, most mothers will abandon mixed-feeding. In theory, HIV-positive women could switch from mixed-feeding to wet-nursing, to heat-treating their expressed breastmilk, to short-term exclusive breastfeeding, or to cup-feeding.

It seems likely, however, that if they are given the choice, many HIV-positive women will switch from mixed-feeding to exclusive bottle-feeding. As Van Esterik (1989) noted, Third World bottles may symbolize death to us, but not to the women involved. Many of them like bottles. Decision-makers in each country will need to determine what options they will support and what training they will give to health workers.

---

# References

Arnold, Lois D. W. 1996. Donor Milk. Appendix to HIV, *Pregnancy and Breastfeeding*, by Edith White. Sandwich, Massachusetts: Health Education Associates.
_____. 1997. How North American donor milk banks operate: Results of a survey, part 1. *Journal of Human Lactation* 13: 159–162.
_____. 1998. HIV and donor milk banks. Available from lactnet@library.ummed.edu; INTERNET, March 4.
Barnett, Tony, and Piers Blaikie. 1992. *AIDS in Africa: Its Present and Future Impact.* New York: Guilford Press.
Becquart, P., et al. 1998. Early postnatal mother-to-child transmission of HIV-1 in Bangui, Central African Republic. Presented at the Fifth Conference on Retroviruses and Opportunistic Infections, Chicago, Illinois, February 1–5.
Belitsky, V. 1989. Children infect mothers in AIDS outbreak at Soviet hospital. *Nature* 337: 493.
Bellamy, Carol. 1998. *The State of the World's Children.* New York: UNICEF.
Bertolli, Jeanne, et al. 1996. Estimating the timing of mother-to-child transmission of human immunodeficiency virus in a breast-feeding population in Kinshasa, Zaire. *Journal of Infectious Diseases* 174: 722–726.
Bobat, R., Moodley Dhayendree, Anna Coutsoudis and Hoosen Coovadia. 1997. Breastfeeding by HIV-1-infected women and outcome in their infants: A cohort study from Durban, South Africa. *AIDS* 11: 1627–1633.
Bobkov, A., et al. 1993. Diversity of HIV-1 V3 domain: A study of the HIV-1 epidemic in the former Soviet Union with different routes of transmission. Presented at the Ninth International Conference on AIDS, Berlin, Germany, June 6–11. Abstract PO-A11-0184.
Bobkov, Aleksei, et al. 1994. Identification of an env G subtype and heterogeneity of HIV-1 strains in the Russian Federation and Belarus. *AIDS* 8: 1649–1655.
Bunce, Matthew. 1997. AIDS gives African mothers cruel choices. *Reuters News Service*, December 14.

Clarkson, T. B., M. S. Anthony and C. L. Hughes. 1995. Estrogenic soybean isoflavones and chronic disease: Risks and benefits. *Trends in Endocrinology and Metabolism* 1: 11–16.

Colebunders, Robert, et al. 1988. Breast-feeding and transmission of HIV. *Lancet* ii: 1487.

Davachi, Farzin. 1994. Pediatric HIV infection in Africa. In *AIDS in Africa*, eds. Max Essex, Souleymane Mboup, Phyllis J. Kanki and Mbowa R. Kalengayi. New York: Raven Press Ltd., pp. 439–462.

De Martino, Maurizio, et al. 1992. HIV-1 transmission through breast milk: Appraisal of the risk according to duration of feeding. *AIDS* 6: 991–997.

Dewey, K. G., and Bo Lonnerdal. 1983. Milk and nutrient intake of breastfed infants from 1 to 6 months: Relation to growth and fatness. *Journal of Pediatric Gastroenterology and Nutrition* 2: 497.

Eglin, R. P., and A. R. Wilkinson 1987. HIV infection and pasteurisation of breastmilk. *Lancet* 329: 1093.

Ehrenkranz, Richard A., and Barbara A. Ackerman. 1986. Metoclopramide effect on faltering milk production by mothers of premature infants. *Pediatrics* 78: 614–620.

Ekpini, E., S. Z. Wiktor and T. Sibailly. 1994. Late postnatal mother-to-child HIV transmission in Abidjan, Côte d'Ivoire. Presented at the Tenth International Conference on AIDS, Yokohama, Japan, August. Abstract 218C.

Ekpini, Ehounou R., et al. 1997. Late postnatal mother-to-child transmission of HIV-1 in Abidjan, Côte d'Ivoire. *Lancet* 349: 1054–1059.

Embree, J., et al. 1993. Delayed seroconversion in infants born to HIV-1 seropositive mothers: Associated factors. Presented at the Ninth International Conference on AIDS, Berlin, Germany, June 6–11. Abstract WS-CO2-4.

Fein, Esther B. 1989. 10 AIDS babies baffling Moscow hospital team. *New York Times*, February 12, p. 22.

Fildes, V. 1986. *Breasts, Bottles and Babies: A History of Infant Feeding*. Edinburgh: Edinburgh University Press.

Fiscus, S. A., et al. 1997. Importance of maternal zidovudine therapy in the reduction of perinatal transmission of HIV. Presented at the Fourth International Conference on Retroviruses and Opportunistic Infections, Washington, D.C., January 22–27.

Fisher, Chloe, and Sally Inch. 1996. Nipple confusion — who is confused? *Journal of Pediatrics* 130: 174.

Geloo, Zarina. 1998. HIV and Breastfeeding: Reigniting an old controversy. Women's Feature Service. *Women's International Net Magazine*. Available at http://www.geocities.com/wellesley/3321/win6d.htm; INTERNET.

Gordon, John E., Ishwari D. Chitkara and John B. Wyon. 1963. Weanling diarrhea. *American Journal of Medical Science* 245: 345–377.

Grant, James P. 1994. *The State of the World's Children*. New York: UNICEF.

Gregson, Simon, Tom Zhuwau, Roy M. Anderson and Stephen K. Chandiwana. 1998. Is there evidence for behavior change in response to AIDS in rural Zimbabwe? *Social Science and Medicine* 46: 321–330.

Greiner, Ted. 1997. Breastfeeding and LAM: Beyond conventional approaches.

Modified from paper presented at the Georgetown University Institute for Reproductive Health End of Project Conference "Bellagio and Beyond," Washington, D.C., May 15–16.

Hawkins, Nancy M., Susan Coffey, Margaret S. Lawson and H. Trevor Delves. 1994. Potential aluminum toxicity in infants fed special infant formula. *Journal of Pediatric Gastroenterology and Nutrition* 19: 377–381.

Ho, T. F., W. C. L. Yip, J. S. H. Tay and H. B. Wong. 1985. Variability in osmolality of home prepared formula milk samples. *Journal of Tropical Pediatrics* 31: 92–94.

Hoover, Kay. 1997. Candidiasis and breastfeeding. Presented at the 1997 International Conference on the Theory and Practice of Human Lactation, Orlando, Florida, January 16–19.

Hwayire, Nyarayi, Hilaria Sibanda and Shellie Phiri. 1996. Consequences facing women living with HIV/AIDS in Zimbabwe. Presented at the Eleventh International Conference on AIDS, Vancouver, Canada, July 7–12. Abstract Tu.D.131.

Infant AIDS Treatment Difficult. 1998. *Associated Press*, March 20.

Ingkaran, N., et. al. 1988. Effect of soy protein on the small bowel mucosa of young infants recovering from acute gastroenteritis. *Journal of Pediatric Gastroenterology and Nutrition* 7: 68–75.

International Code of Marketing of Breastmilk Substitutes. 1981. *World Health Assembly Resolution 34.22*, May.

International News. 1996. *Baby Milk Action News*, March 18.

Irvine, Cliff, Mike Fitzpatrick, Iain Robertson and David Woodhams. 1995. The potential adverse effects of soybean phytoestrogens in infant feeding. *New Zealand Medical Journal* 108: 208–209.

Irvine, C. H., M. G. Fitzpatrick and S. L. Alexander. 1998. Phytoestrogens in soy-based infant foods: Concentrations' daily intake and possible biological effects. *Proceedings of the Society for Experimental Biology and Medicine* 217: 247–253.

John, Grace. 1998. Personal communication to author.

Karlsson, Katrina, et al. 1997. Late postnatal transmission of human immunodeficiency virus type 1 infection from mothers to infants in Dar es Salaam, Tanzania. *Pediatric Infectious Disease Journal* 16: 963–967.

Keogh, P., et al. 1994. The social impact of HIV infection on women in Kigali, Rwanda: A prospective study. *Social Science and Medicine* 38 (8): 1047–1053.

Kline, M. W., et. al. 1996. Oral manifestations and microflora of infants and children with vertical human immunodeficiency virus (HIV) infection. Presented at the Eleventh International Conference on AIDS, Vancouver, Canada, July 7–12. Abstract We.B.3304.

Krivine, A., S. Le Bourdelles, G. Firtion and P. Lebon. 1997. Viral kinetics in HIV-1 perinatal infection. *Lancet* 350: 493.

La Leche League International. 1997. *Role of Mother's Milk in HIV Transmission Remains Unclear*. Schaumburg, Illinois: La Leche League International.

Lallemant, Marc, Sophie Le Coeur, Donald Shepard and Richard Marlink. 1996. Preventing mother-to-child HIV transmission in resource-poor countries: A cost effectiveness perspective. Presented at the Eleventh International Conference on AIDS, Vancouver, Canada, July 7-12. Abstract Th.C.4822.

Lang, Sandra, Clive J. Lawrence and Richard L'E Orme. 1994. Cup feeding: An alternative method of infant feeding. *Archives of Disease in Childhood* 71: 365–369.

Latham, Michael C., K. Okoth Agunda and Terry Elliot. 1988. Infant feeding in Nairobi, Kenya. In *Feeding Infants in Four Societies*, eds. Beverly Winikoff, Mary Ann Castle, Virginia Hight Laukaran. New York: Greenwood Press, pp. 67–94.

Lawrence, Ruth A. 1989. *Breastfeeding; A Guide for the Medical Profession*, Third Edition. St. Louis: C.V. Mosby Company.

Lonnerdal, B., et al. 1989. Inhibitory effects of phytic acid and other inositol phosphates on zinc and calcium absorption in suckling rats. *Journal of Nutrition* 119: 211–214.

Mansergh, Gordon, et al. 1996. Cost effectiveness of short-course zidovudine to prevent perinatal HIV type 1 infection in a sub–Saharan African developing country setting. *Journal of the American Medical Association* 276: 149.

National Alliance for Breastfeeding Advocacy in US. 1997. *HIV and Infant Feeding.* Weston, Massachusetts: NABA.

Narayanan, Indira, K. Prakash, N. S. Murthy and V. V. Gujral. 1984. Randomized controlled trial of effect of raw and holder pasteurised human milk and formula supplements on incidence of neonatal infection. *Lancet* 323: 1111–1113.

Nduati, Ruth W., Grace C. John and J. Kreiss. 1994. Postnatal transmission of HIV-1 through pooled breast milk. *Lancet* 344: 1432.

Nicoll, Angus, and Marie-Louise Newell. 1996. Preventing perinatal transmission of HIV: The effect of breast-feeding (letter). *Journal of the American Medical Association* 276: 1552

Nutrition Division of the Uganda Ministry of Health, Child Health and Development Center of Makerere University and Wellstart International. 1994. *Breastfeeding in Uganda: Beliefs and Practices.*Washington, D.C.: USAID.

Orloff, S. L., et al. 1993. Inactivation of human immunodeficiency virus type 1 in human milk: Effects of intrinsic factors in human milk and of pasteurization. *Journal of Human Lactation* 9: 13–17.

Perez-Gil, Sara Elena. 1996. Breastfeeding and Maternal Employment. In *Exclusive Breastfeeding Promotion*. Washington, D.C.: USAID.

Poprovsky, V. V., et al. 1991. HIV-transmission in the USSR. Presented at the Seventh International Conference on AIDS, Florence, Italy, June 16–21. Abstract WC 3056.

Prescott, Nicholas, et al. 1996. Formulating rational use of anti-retrovirals in Thailand. Presented at the Eleventh International Conference on AIDS, Vancouver, Canada, July 7–12. Abstract Mo.B.533.

Raphael, Dana. 1973. *The Tender Gift: Breastfeeding*. Englewood Cliffs, New Jersey: Prentice Hall.

Remnick, D. 1989. Unwashed needles infect 27 infants with AIDS. *Washington Post*, January 29, p. A31.

Rubini, N. P., et al. 1994. Risks of bottle-feeding infants born to HIV-infected mothers from low-income families in Rio de Janeiro. Presented at the Tenth International Conference on AIDS, Yokohama, Japan, August 7–12. Abstract PCO158.

Ruff, A., et al. 1994. Excretion of zidovudine (ZDV) in human breast milk. Presented at the Interscientific Conference on Antimicrobial Agents and Chemotherapy, October.

Saadeh, Randa J., Miriam H. Labbok, Kristin A. Cooney and Peggy Koniz-Booher, eds. 1993. *Breast-feeding: The Technical Basis for Action.* Geneva, Switzerland: World Health Organization.

Setchell, K. D., L. Zimmer-Nechemias, J. Cai and J. E. Heubi. 1997. Exposure of infants to phyto-estrogens from soy-based infant formula. *Lancet* 350: 23–27.

Söderlund, Neil, et al. 1998. Breast or bottle? A cost-effectiveness evaluation of formula feeding for the prevention of postnatal transmission of HIV in an urban South African setting. Presented at the Twelfth World AIDS Conference, Geneva, Switzerland, June 28–July 3. Abstract 24124.

Springer, Skadi. 1997. Human milk banking in Germany. *Journal of Human Lactation* 13: 65–68.

UNAIDS Joint United Nations Programme on HIV/AIDS. 1996. HIV and Infant Feeding: An Interim Statement. *Weekly Epidemiological Record* 71: 289–291.

_____. 1997a. *HIV and Infant Feeding.* A Policy Statement. Geneva, Switzerland: UNAIDS.

_____. 1997b. *Report on the Global HIV/AIDS Epidemic.* Geneva, Switzerland: UNAIDS.

_____. 1998. International meeting calls for concerted action to prevent mother-to-child transmission of HIV. Press release, Geneva, Switzerland, March 24.

UNICEF. 1998. *New HIV/AIDS Treatment Will Save Thousands of Children.* New York: UNICEF, March 26.

UNICEF, UNAIDS, and the World Health Organization. 1998a. *HIV and Infant Feeding: Guidelines for decision-makers.* Geneva, Switzerland: World Health Organization.

UNICEF, UNAIDS, and the World Health Organization. 1998b. *HIV and Infant Feeding: A Guide for Health Care Managers and Supervisors.* Geneva, Switzerland: World Health Organization.

Urban, Mike. 1997. Attitudes and practices of infant feeding in HIV-1 infected women in Soweto. Presented at the Conference on Affordable Options for the Prevention of Mother-to-child Transmission of HIV-1, Johannesburg, South Africa, November 19–20.

Van Esterik, Penny. 1989. *Beyond the Breast-Bottle Controversy.* New Brunswick, New Jersey: Rutgers University Press.

Wallingford, J. C., and J. S. McDougal. 1993. Inactivation of human immunodeficiency virus type 1 in human milk: Effects of intrinsic factors in human milk and of pasteurization. *Journal of Human Lactation* 9: 13–17.

Welbourn, H. F., and G. De Beer. 1964. Trial of a kit for artificial feeding in tropical village homes. *Journal of Tropical Medicine and Hygiene* 67: 155.

Wellstart Intl. Expanded Promotion of Breastfeeding Program. 1994. *Final Report of Program in Rwanda, March 1992–April 1994.* Washington, D.C.: USAID.

Wiktor, Stefan Z. 1997. Trial in Côte d'Ivoire. Presented at the Tenth Conference on HIV and STDs in Africa, Abidjan, Côte d'Ivoire, December 7–11.

Woods, Dave. 1997. A national dried milk formula. Presented at the Conference on Affordable Options for the Prevention of Mother-to-child Transmission of HIV-1, Johannesburg, South Africa, November 19–20.

World Alliance for Breastfeeding Action. Undated Discussion Paper. *Expressing Ourselves: Breast Pumps*. Penang, Malaysia: WABA.

World Health Organization, UNAIDS and UNICEF. 1998. *Technical Consultation on HIV and Infant Feeding, Geneva, Switzerland, April 20–22*. Conclusions.

Ziemer, Mary, Diane M. Cooper and Joseph G. Pigeon. 1995. Evaluation of a dressing to reduce nipple pain and improve nipple skin condition in breast-feeding women. *Nursing Research* 44: 347–351.

Zoppi, G., et al. 1983. Diet and antibody responses to vaccinations in healthy infants. *Lancet* ii: 11–14.

Zoppi, G., et al. 1989. Response to RIT 4237 oral rotavirus vaccine in human milk, adapted and soy formula-fed infants. *Acta Paediatrica Scandanavia* 78: 759–762.

CHAPTER TEN

Issues and
Recommendations
for Policy Makers

Should the world community offer HIV-positive mothers information about the risks and benefits of breastfeeding and provide them with feeding alternatives if they choose not to nurse? Yes, of course it should. It is the right thing to do. UNAIDS clinical research specialist Joseph Saba (1997) said that we do not want the world to say to us later that we knew about this situation (HIV and breastfeeding) but did nothing.

This chapter addresses issues relating to the decisions public health officials will need to consider in setting policies about HIV and infant feeding. These include concerns about human rights, untested women and costs; regard for industrialized, intermediate and resource-poor countries; and the broader interest in protecting breastfeeding. The chapter closes with recommendations.

## Governments Set Policy

It is the responsibility of the public health officials of each nation to set policy based on the country's traditions, economic position, and patterns of HIV prevalence, child mortality and infant feeding. International and regional health groups can make recommendations, but governments need to implement policies. For example, it was the *recommendation* of those attending the November 1997 meeting of eleven Latin American countries that HIV-infected mothers should not breastfeed (Johnson 1997). They also concluded that HIV-positive women should be told about the risk of transmission via breastfeeding even when alternatives were not provided (Izazola-Licea 1998). But it is up to each Latin American government to decide whether to provide AZT or alternatives to breastfeeding. In an effort to assist government officials, UNICEF, UNAIDS and the WHO issued guidelines for decision makers (1998a) and for health care managers and supervisors (1998b), who can now consider these recommendations in deciding what policies best fit their own countries.

Public health officials would be wise to invite the participation of women's groups, AIDS groups and other NGOs in policy debates, as collaborative efforts might bring about compliance among people who mistrust government. Moreover, some African women have asserted that they must participate in the political process when the health care of ordinary citizens is at issue: "African women are now asserting that it is the vulnerability of the state that renders it incapable of addressing their needs, and their major responsibility must be to participate in local, public and political processes" (Mikell 1997:32).

## *Three Areas Where Decisions Need to Be Made*

Those who set policy will need to establish infant-feeding guidelines instructing health workers: (1) how to advise tested HIV-positive women, (2) what to say during the counseling sessions designed to precede HIV testing, and (3) what to tell untested women.

What to say to women who have already tested HIV-positive appears most clean-cut. The recommended policy is that these women be counseled about the risks and benefits of breastfeeding, informed of other methods of infant-feeding and allowed to make their own informed decisions.

The second issue relates to what health workers will say in the counseling sessions designed to precede HIV testing. Decision-makers may want the counselors to motivate women to accept testing by telling them it will enable them to make an informed decision about infant-feeding, and also about treatment with any available antiretroviral drugs.

Most challenging will be the third issue. What should health workers say to the huge majority of women who cannot or will not be tested? These are the millions of women whose feeding practices will greatly affect child mortality rates in the next few years.

Policy-makers could decide to follow the guidelines issued by UNAIDS, UNICEF and the World Health Organization (1998), which recommended that, for untested women, breastfeeding be protected, promoted and supported. Dr. Felicity Savage-King (1998) of the WHO recommended that health workers not discuss replacement-feeding unless the women know and accept their HIV status. This suggests that health workers would simply keep quiet about HIV when they discuss infant-feeding advice with untested women. They would not mention, for example, the fact that short-term breastfeeding may be a safer alternative than long-term breastfeeding.

Decision-makers could argue that public health calculations support a policy of not mentioning HIV transmission via breastmilk, lest the conversation raise doubts in the minds of untested women. But while a policy of silence may be practical for areas where the grapevine has not yet spread hearsay about breastmilk and HIV, it will not address the concerns of women who have already heard the rumors. If untested (but HIV-infected) women end up breastfeeding — or feeding their babies overdiluted formula out of fear — the policy of keeping mum is unlikely to decrease rising child mortality rates.

## Considering Spillover

The 1998 guidelines for health care managers and supervisors recommend that workers deciding to procure and distribute commercial infant formula take measures to prevent spillover (UNICEF/UNAIDS/WHO 1998a:23). Spillover refers to HIV-negative and untested women avoiding breastfeeding because of fears about HIV. Health workers are supposed to prevent spillover by emphasizing the benefits of breastfeeding and the dangers of artificial feeding, by restricting information about formula and by keeping formula out of sight. Health care managers are supposed to ensure that health workers know their responsibilities under the Code and strengthen UNICEF's Baby Friendly Hospital Initiative.

This advice, however, seems based on two questionable assumptions — that spillover is caused by formula distribution and that spillover can be prevented by following the same old interventions that did not succeed previously in getting women to feed as recommended. There is no evidence that spillover is caused by formula distribution. Formula availability is likely to exacerbate the trend away from breastfeeding, but spillover has occurred for years. There was no formula dispensed when women were afraid to breastfeed in Zaire in 1988, in Zambia in 1991, and in Zimbabwe in 1998. It wasn't formula; it was fear of AIDS. Berer (1993:84) pointed out that African women had already tended not to breastfeed. But now the trend will grow because of women's "fears that they may have HIV, their refusal to be tested because they really do not want to know, and now their fear of transmitting HIV to their infants."

Nor is there any evidence to support the hope that spillover can be prevented by same old interventions (the telling of the benefits of breastfeeding, the telling of the dangers of artificial feeding, the restriction of formula, and the appeal to the Code and to Baby Friendly). There is no evidence that these measures restored exclusive breastfeeding, even in the pre-AIDS era, during which time women believed that breastmilk was the best food for their babies. Mothers may not have been able, or willing, to nurse as often as recommended (breastfeeding exclusively entails nursing about ten times a day), despite believing that breast was best. Now that women in some areas associate breastfeeding with transmission of AIDS (Ighogboja 1995, Wellstart 1994, Urban 1997, Gregson 1998), it seems much less likely that health workers will be able to use the old interventions to prevent spillover.

## Human Rights and Infant Feeding

The HIV/AIDS pandemic may have had one silver lining, as it intensified interest in the connection between human rights and public health and emphasized that decisions should be made in accordance with ethical concerns and human rights principles. Gostin and Lazzarini (1997) note how human rights concerns relate to infant feeding policies in developing countries. They argue that the state has a heavy burden to ensure that children thrive, and contend that if a state recommends HIV-infected mothers forego breastfeeding, it has an obligation to provide clean water, formula and health education.

The UNAIDS/UNICEF/WHO 1996-1997 interim policy statement declared that all women, irrespective of HIV status, have the right both to determine the course of their reproductive health and to have access to information. It does not specify, however, which information untested women have a right to access. That will be up to decision-makers in each country.

The Universal Declaration of Human Rights (1948) affirmed the right to life and the right to access to information. This statement, like the Convention on the Rights of the Child (1989), declared that in all actions concerning children, the child's best interests should be a primary consideration. Whether a child's right not to ingest virus-laden breastmilk is in conflict with a woman's right to breastfeed (to conceal seropositivity) could be debated. But it is hard to imagine that encouraging an HIV-positive woman to use replacement-feeding without regard to her assessment of personal circumstances would be in her child's best interests. Children's survival under conditions of poverty is closely related to their mothers' survival. If, for instance, a woman's fears are realized and her male partner throws her out for being infected, her baby may experience risks greater than the one associated with ingestion of virus-laden breastmilk.

The Second International Convention on HIV/AIDS and Human Rights, which met in Geneva in 1996, declared that all people had the right to freely receive and impart information, including HIV-related prevention information. Information about breastmilk and HIV is important prevention information, especially in high prevalence areas.

Although knowing one's HIV status is crucial in making an informed infant-feeding decision, none of the human rights declarations have a footnote saying that women give up their right to access to information if they are unable or unwilling to undergo HIV testing. Neither do the human rights declarations say that untested people should be denied access to general HIV prevention information. Untested people are, quite to the contrary, supposed to be given HIV prevention information about sexual contacts, needle-sharing, and other means of contracting the virus. Finally, none of the human rights declarations say that untested Third World women make up a special subcategory of people for whom HIV prevention information should be withheld, as others deem appropriate.

## Making the Case for Telling All Pregnant Women About HIV

Many pregnant women live in areas where HIV testing will become available. Health workers in these high prevalence areas could tell all pregnant women that HIV-infected females can reduce risk of mother-to-child transmission by avoiding breastfeeding, especially partial prolonged breastfeeding. Health workers could tell all pregnant women that if they are tested they will know the safest way to feed their baby. Gostin and Lazzarini (1997:153) suggest that it is a realistic alternative to provide women with full information as prelude to an offer for testing: "The Ministry (of Health) could advise women of the risk of HIV transmission through breast-feeding and offer to test them on a confidential and voluntary basis."

If antiretroviral drugs such as AZT become available, health workers could be trained to inform all pregnant women of the drugs' effectiveness. Health workers could help all pregnant women to understand the issues in mother-to-child HIV transmission, regardless of whether each individual chooses to be tested, to learn the results of her HIV test, to disclose seropositivity, to take AZT, or to breastfeed.

Restricting information about breastmilk-related transmission for women who have already tested HIV-positive keeps important information from everyone. The Second International Consultation on AIDS has noted that governments may impose restrictions on some rights, to meet important goals such as public health, if they pass laws. A government could assert that withholding information about HIV transmission via breastmilk will achieve lower overall child mortality rates by minimizing fear-driven "irrational" breastfeeding avoidance. No government has passed a law declaring that public health goals dictate that information about HIV and breastmilk be withheld from untested women.

Where HIV testing and counseling programs are either unavailable, despite high HIV prevalence, information about mother-to-child HIV transmission could be dispensed in other prenatal contacts. HIV prevention information is as relevant to child survival as Code-required counseling on the difficulty in reversing the decision not to breastfeed. If it is decided that women in high prevalence areas should know that their breastmilk supply will dwindle if they don't breastfeed regularly, all women (tested or not) should be made aware that the breastmilk of infected women can transmit HIV.

An additional argument in favor of giving untested pregnant women information about risks and benefits is that, in some areas, health workers could protect breastfeeding by clearing up misconceptions. Many women in Capetown, South Africa, for instance, incorrectly assumed that all babies breastfed by HIV-infected mothers would become infected (Kuhn 1997). Baker (1991) noted that many women in Zambia believed breastfeeding to be dangerous. Where radio and "street radio" give women unbalanced information, health workers can give a more balanced view.

Another reason why decision makers should have health workers discuss HIV with all pregnant women in high prevalence areas is that doing so might maintain confidence in the health care system. If the health care system is seen as ignoring the problem of breastmilk transmission of HIV, then there may be a loss of confidence in the system, which might have a negative impact on other important interventions (Nduati 1998).

## The Tension Between Protecting Breastfeeding and Adapting to HIV

Debates about infant-feeding education and HIV — like other AIDS issues — have the potential to bring out diametrically opposing points of view. For example, Jonathan Mann, founding director of the WHO's Global Programme on AIDS, sparked debate when he said, "The failure to proceed expeditiously with field trials of available AIDS vaccine candidates constitutes unethical practice and violates human rights of Americans" (Mann 1998). Those who took exception to Mann's point of view cited traditional scientific methodology. The question of the appropriate pace of AIDS vaccine trials, then, pits two camps against each other. Likewise, the policy of keeping HIV-breastmilk information from millions of untested pregnant women is adamantly opposed by those who believe it to be a human rights violation and steadfastly supported by others who see it as sound breastfeeding protectionism.

Nduati (1998) noted that finding a solution to various problems has been argued as a "pre-condition for implementing a programme to prevent breastmilk transmission of HIV in resource-poor settings." And the problems believed most in need of solution — such as the growing number of orphans, the issue of women's confidentiality, the need to preserve gains in breastfeeding promotion efforts — are daunting. Moreover, as Jonathan Mann argues, anything that "creates an unreasonable barrier to progress" is unethical.

A government that chooses the protection of breastfeeding as the number one priority may decide that health workers should mention breastmilk-related transmission only to tested HIV-positive women or to women who are being urged to accept testing. They would say nothing to women who are unwilling or unable to undergo HIV testing.

A government that chooses the protection of breastfeeding as the number one priority may want health workers to continue to deliberately portray formula feeding or bottle-feeding as negative. A rural postnatal clinic on an island in the Grenadines, West Indies, had a large hand-lettered poster that read, "Any mother found bottlefeeding her baby will not be treated at this clinic" (Payne 1997). Health workers in Yemen developed a poster that depicted baby bottles as dangerous weapons (Greiner 1993).

A government that chooses the protection of breastfeeding as the number one priority may put pressure on HIV-positive women to cup-feed rather than bottle-feed. Ensuring that mothers are taught to use cups is considered a practice designed to prevent the spillover effect (UNICEF/UNAIDS/WHO 1998).

A government that chooses the protection of breastfeeding as the number one priority may not be interested in using camouflage strategies to destigmatize formula-feeding. In describing feasibility studies in Haiti, Coreil (1998) reported how women and health workers reacted to the idea of a bottle-feeding trial for HIV-infected women. She noted that formula-feeding can announce a woman's seropositivity and discussed the idea of a camouflage strategy. In a previous camouflage strategy, researchers invited some HIV-negative mothers and babies to a clinic for AIDS studies that was called, simply and misleadingly, "Breastfeeding Clinic." To camouflage formula-feeding, health care workers might likewise include uninfected women. But including uninfected women in formula-feeding trials could be seen as undermining breastfeeding promotion efforts. As Coreil and others have noted, breastfeeding is already undermined if women think that medical personnel endorse bottle-feeding.

## Primary Infections During Breastfeeding

As policy makers decide whether their guidelines will lean more heavily toward either protecting breastfeeding or destigmatizing replacement-feeding, they will also need to decide what to say about seroconverting breastfeeding women. In 1997, the Appropriate Health Resources and Technologies and Action Group (AHRTAG) published a booklet in which it recommended ways health workers in resource-poor countries might talk to (largely untested) pregnant women about infant feeding. In the report, AHRTAG wrote, "It is very

important for health workers to explain about the increased risk of passing
HIV to the baby if she becomes infected while she is breastfeeding and to advise
about preventing infection."

But if the protection of breastfeeding is seen as the number one priority,
then policy makers may choose not to have health workers warn women of
the dangers of breastfeeding during seroconversion, lest the information
undermine breastfeeding promotion efforts. What if it leaves the impression
that no woman with a sexual partner is safe enough to breastfeed? What if a
woman feels that her male partner will not put up with condoms (male or
female)? Against this, one might argue that HIV-negative and untested women
have the right to the information, that their understanding may motivate them
to remain uninfected, and that health workers are in no position to assess the
sexual habits of women's male partners.

## The Need to Study Breastfeeding Avoidance

Although there is much angst over fear-driven breastfeeding avoidance
(the so-called spillover effect), the phenomenon has not been researched.
Dr. Nils Daulaire of the U.S. Agency for International Development said, "Doctors must figure out how to curb nursing by HIV-infected mothers without
harming the bigger message" (Infant AIDS Treatment 1998). When doctors
want to figure out something, they generally commission research. To fail to
conduct research on fear-driven breastfeeding avoidance is to be remiss. To
continue to focus on formula company monitoring — to the exclusion of other
aspects of breastfeeding protectionism — seems a bit like rearranging deck
chairs on the Titanic.

If efforts were directed toward the active study of fear-driven breastfeeding avoidance, then breastfeeding protectionism in the late 1990s might
offer more insight. The ten-country demonstration project UNICEF will man-
age, as well as other pilot projects, could study this issue. If social scientists,
psychologists and anthropologists were included, much could be learned about
the mothers' knowledge, attitudes, beliefs and practices (KABP). Tested and
untested women and other members of their families could be invited to participate in focus groups. Community participation has been called a "must"
for HIV/AIDS prevention in Africa (CAFOD 1998). Participatory research methods might uncover specific local beliefs, which could then be incorporated
into infant feeding discussions with local pregnant women.

The topic of breastfeeding avoidance — in the broadest sense — could be
studied using KABP evaluations. In fact, at least one breastfeeding anthropologist has already studied the phenomenon of breastfeeding avoidance (unrelated to HIV). Vanessa Maher argues that the custom of breastfeeding avoidance should be examined in cultural terms, not in the positivist terms of the

medical model, which has not effectively dealt with the "problem" of breast-feeding. Maher (1995:175) writes, "The 'medical model' as regards breast-feeding appears to belong to an outdated positivist tradition, which is anthropologically interesting but highly dangerous if it is to inform policies towards women."

Health workers have for years been trained in the medical model (breast is best, tell all women to breastfeed). These health workers are likely to find it extremely challenging to talk women out of fear-driven breastfeeding avoidance. As yet, there are no guidelines that might help a counselor allay a woman's fear that her promiscuous male partner might infect her, and that she in turn might infect her breastfeeding baby.

Perhaps there is an approach that health workers can use in talking to fearful women. Perhaps not. Regardless, it is time to devote serious study to fear-driven breastfeeding avoidance. Health workers were not able to talk most women out of their "irrational" reluctance to feed colostrum or "bad" milk even before hard science found a reason for their behavior. Workers were not able to convince most women to breastfeed exclusively for four to six months even when mothers believed that it was the best way to feed their baby.

If researchers choose to study fear-driven breastfeeding avoidance, they may find it useful to do so within the broader context of general breastfeeding avoidance. Do they agree with Maher's contention that a new, cultural perspective is warranted? Do they agree that overworked, undersupported, underfed women are rational in trying to offload some of the burden of infant-feeding that they have been bearing alone from the limited resources of their own bodies? Do they agree that societies have chosen not to lighten women's burdens in such a way as to foster exclusive breastfeeding? Finally, do they agree that women generally do the best that they can for their babies, as well as themselves?

## The Unsuccessful Use of Exhortations

If HIV-infant feeding policy debates do not expand to include larger issues, it seems unlikely that they will succeed in convincing all women to feed according to tested HIV status. Policies that focus on exhortations — such as Use condoms consistently! Breastfeed exclusively! and Feed your baby according to your tested HIV status! — seem especially unlikely to succeed. Policies must go beyond simple goading and be informed by more than just the positivist medical model.

Policy makers need to broaden their approach to address the barriers to each component in a desired policy. It is not enough to say that women should choose to undergo HIV testing. Women's reluctance to be screened, as well as other barriers to testing, must be understood. It is not enough to say that HIV-positive women should be allowed to make informed choices about formula-feeding. Steps must be taken to destigmatize replacement feeding as a sign of seropositivity.

It is not enough to say that HIV-negative women should breastfeed exclusively. Policy makers need to acknowledge the fear that is driving uninfected women away from breastfeeding. Policy makers need also to recognize that women's manifold responsibilities are preventing exclusive breastfeeding, and that societies are not lightening women's burdens.

Policy makers need to decide whether they wish to change the fact that most babies of untested HIV-infected mothers are receiving partial prolonged breastfeeding. Does the protection of breastfeeding justify not telling untested women in high prevalence areas that partial prolonged breastfeeding is the worst infant feeding method for children of HIV-infected women? Does lack of disclosure discriminate against women's right to access information and children's right to life? If nothing is said about the risks and benefits of partial prolonged breastfeeding, then child mortality rates in high prevalence areas are likely to continue to rise. Then what?

## Issues for Industrialized and Intermediate Countries

Decision-makers in industrialized and intermediate countries, as well as those in resource-poor countries, will need to balance funding for HIV/AIDS interventions with competing health needs. The higher the prevalence rates, the more cost effective are funding initiatives for HIV testing, for antiretroviral drugs and for formula.

Decision-makers also need to discuss whether they will recommend that HIV be routinely mentioned in sessions with pregnant women. Funding antiretrovirals without also explaining the benefit of testing seems like a poor use of financial resources. A report from San Francisco made evident that even in the United States, where policy supports free antiretroviral drug therapy for pregnant HIV-positive women, education lags behind. Only 24 percent of HIV-positive women knew that medication could reduce the risk of mother-to-child HIV transmission (Carusi 1998). Women who do not understand how to reduce mother-to-child transmission are less likely to accept HIV testing.

Bertolli reported that as of 1996 some HIV-positive U.S. women, largely those whose seropositivity had not been identified during pregnancy, were still breastfeeding. Tess (1997) communicated from Brazil that some HIV-positive women, unaware of their HIV status, were breastfeeding. Urban (1997) noted that women who received only one counseling session were less likely to understand HIV transmission via breastfeeding.

In a report about data collected in 1995, Bertolli (1998) reported that some U.S. children of HIV-positive women were not receiving the prescribed treatment. While 81 percent of 1100 HIV-exposed children received at least some component of antiretroviral drug therapy, only 53 percent received the full drug regimen. The most common reasons were lack of early prenatal care and refusal of treatment. Although the study was conducted in 1995, and a larger percentage of children are now likely to receive full treatment, the lack of access to early prenatal care is still apparent.

Even in industrialized countries, pediatric AIDS may be the first sign of maternal HIV disease. Goldstein and Sever (1996) described the situation for 25 of the HIV-positive children they treated in the United States:

> To our discomfort and horror, 9 of these patients first became aware of their HIV status by having a prior child admitted to the Children's National Medical Center with an AIDS-defining illness. Six of these children died. Like the canaries carried by coal miners in the previous century whose death would portend the presence of lethal gases, these children are the unfortunate sentinels of undiagnosed HIV infection.

Since the time of that report, HIV testing of pregnant women in the United States has become more common, although not universal. In many countries babies or older children with AIDS–defining illnesses are still the "unfortunate sentinels" of maternal HIV infection.

## Routine Mention of HIV

Two states in the United States have required that their public health workers routinely mention HIV to all pregnant clients, tested or not. Since people have the right to keep their seropositivity confidential, these health workers do not ask women about their HIV status. From the 1995 Policy and Procedure Manual of the New Jersey Department of Health WIC Services comes this statement:

> In the first nutrition education contact and during the prenatal breast-feeding class, all women must be provided with the following information: a.) the Department of Health recommends HIV testing of all pregnant women, b.) women should know their HIV status before deciding to breastfeed because there is a risk of passing HIV through breastmilk, and c.) women who are HIV-positive should not breastfeed.

The *New York State Department of Health Policy on Breastfeeding and HIV* (1991) noted that health care providers should not assume any woman's HIV status based on perceived or self-reported risk factors. Instead, they should advise all women of the risk of HIV transmission to their infants. Over time, women in New York State have become increasingly open about discussing their HIV status, although some still choose not to disclose it. Public health workers provide all pregnant women with the same basic information. The New York policy statement advises,

> If the woman is known to be HIV-negative, breastfeeding should be encouraged. It is essential to stress HIV risk reduction to all HIV-negative women who choose to breastfeed since HIV-infection may be transmitted more efficiently through breastmilk during the period right after infection.

Statistics indicate no "spillover" has resulted from the routine disclosure of breastmilk transmission risks. In fact, breastfeeding rates in New York (Barber 1998) and in New Jersey (Rotundo 1998) have gone up consistently since the policies were instituted,

An additional argument could be made that talking about HIV will help to normalize conversation about it. The women who are currently public health clients will consciously or unconsciously decide what to say to their children on the subject. It will not help the next generation to avoid the virus if their mothers are encouraged in the attitude that HIV/AIDS is off limits in conversation.

## The Need for Training

Health workers in all countries will clearly need training about HIV/AIDS. Those who deal with pregnant women require specific training and need to have misconceptions clarified. They need also to be trained to see that they cannot omit discussion of HIV, even among women they believe to be low risk; heterosexual sex is the most common route of HIV infection among women. Health workers who make assumptions about which women are HIV-infected are often wrong. A prospective study in inner-city Baltimore, Maryland, found that screening based on women's admitting risk factors was not effective. Only 57 percent of HIV-infected women would have been identified, as 43 percent denied high-risk behavior (Barbacci 1991). Coplan (1995) reported that relying on obtaining a history of risk-related behavior before performing HIV testing identified fewer than half of all HIV-infected pregnant or childbearing women. He suggested that because the majority of babies in his area were white and did not fit the racial stereotypic pattern, physicians made the assumption that they were uninfected. Thus 56 percent of HIV-positive children were not identified.

Health workers need to understand their country's policies about infant-feeding advice for tested HIV-positive women, for women receiving pretest counseling and for untested women. They need to understand the risk of transmission via breastmilk for infected women and the risk of transmission by HIV-negative women who later become infected. Perhaps, above all, health workers will need help adjusting to the transition from the era of "Breast is Best" to the era of informed choice.

Policy recommendations will vary according to seroprevalence and degree of development, but some suggestions apply to all countries.

## Recommendations for All Countries

- Emphasize measures that help women avoid becoming HIV-infected. Include male partners in dialogues.
- Expand policy debates to include more representatives from women's groups, AIDS groups, church groups, breastfeeding advocacy groups and other NGOs.
- Provide health workers with training about HIV/AIDS.
- Emphasize to health workers the importance of a woman's right to keep her HIV status confidential, even in societies where people typically know details of other people's lives — where shared confidentiality may be the best option.
- Clarify that "counseling" does not mean telling people what to do.
- Provide babies of informed HIV-positive mothers with accessible replacement-feeding, including affordable infant formula.
- Teach mothers to replacement-feed safely.
- Give HIV-positive mothers information about risks and benefits of cup-feeding and bottle-feeding, allowing them to make an informed choice. Provide practical information about cleaning to mothers who choose to bottle-feed.
- Continue to protect, promote and support breastfeeding in ways that are based on research dialogue rather than on advocacy dialogue. Prioritize breastfeeding efforts to focus first on support for new mothers and last on promotion efforts. Continue to protect breastfeeding, but do more than monitor the formula companies; address additionally the issues of overwork/undersupport and fear-driven breastfeeding avoidance.
- Foster the establishment of support networks for both breastfeeding and nonbreastfeeding women, and refer mothers to them. Remind health workers that peer support is more effective than lecturing.
- Help women control their own fertility by making available contraceptives to women who want them.

## Additional Recommendations for Resource-Poor Countries with High Seroprevalence

• Seek financial support from international agencies, donor nations and foundations, NGOs, pharmaceutical companies, formula manufacturers and other groups to make available voluntary testing and counseling programs, affordable antiretroviral drugs and low-priced infant formula.
• Involve women's groups, AIDS groups and other NGOs to work with the health ministry of each country to set up councils to support safe replacement-feeding, including formula feeding. Encourage dialogue and debate before setting policies over specific issues such as the advantages and disadvantages of making formula a prescription-only item.
• Provide training and support for health workers. Help them to deal with their own concerns, including those surrounding the transition from "Breast is Best" to informed choice. Convince counselors of the need to teach mothers about safe replacement feeding, providing them with clear guidelines on what to say to tested and untested women.
• Have health workers give all pregnant women information about the benefits of knowing their HIV status, including the fact that such knowledge allows women to make informed infant-feeding decisions. Have health workers allow all women access to the information that breastmilk from HIV-infected mothers can transmit HIV. Allow all women access to the information that HIV-negative women who become infected while breastfeeding have a substantial risk of infecting their babies at the breast.
• If antiretroviral drugs are available, have health workers tell all pregnant women that another reason for knowing one's HIV status is that only tested HIV-positive mothers will be granted access to drugs that protect their unborn babies.
• Instruct health workers in the need to teach HIV-positive mothers how to maximize the safety of replacement feeding, including use of formula or modified animal milks and support for mothers to make an informed choice for cup or bottle-feeding.
• Destigmatize formula-feeding and bottle-feeding.

## Additional Recommendations for Industrialized and Intermediate Countries with High Seroprevalence

• Make available for all pregnant women voluntary HIV testing and counseling programs. For those who test positive, make available antiretroviral drug therapy (of an affordable duration) and low-priced infant formula.
• In pretest counseling and in general prenatal contacts, inform all pregnant women of the benefits of being tested. Give women specific information

about available options (such as antiretroviral drug therapy, cesarean delivery and formula feeding).
- Tell all women, tested or not, that babies of HIV-infected mothers can almost always be protected from infection when women are tested and then treated with antiretroviral drugs and when they avoid breastfeeding.

## Additional Recommendations for Manufacturers of Antiretroviral Drugs and Infant Formula

- Continue to cooperate in the provision of affordable antiretroviral drugs and infant formula to research teams and agencies that will distribute them to HIV-positive people.
- Manufacturers of drugs should consider lowering prices, not just for the duration of a woman's pregnancy, but for extended use and for all people.
- Manufacturers of infant formula should consider lowering their prices and should also cooperate with health officials in making affordable formula available to babies of HIV-positive women for as long as they need it, generally for six months. Manufacturers should also take the necessary action to ensure that their conduct at every level conforms to the principles and aim of the Code.

## Additional Recommendations for Researchers and Policy Makers

- Amend the Code to reflect the fact that babies of HIV-infected mothers have a medical need for breastmilk substitutes and that all women have a right to access not only information about the risks and benefits of breastfeeding but about other methods of infant feeding as well.
- Conduct additional research, both quantitative and participatory, and perform KABP evaluations to better understand people's knowledge, attitudes, beliefs, and practices. Study fear-driven breastfeeding avoidance and HIV testing avoidance within the broader context of women's lives (that is, considering such factors as lack of autonomy, gender inequality and poverty).
- Encourage cooperation between local and international researchers to learn how to better present information about infant-feeding among women who know that breastmilk can transmit HIV. Develop innovative approaches in presenting the benefits of breastfeeding to encourage non-infected women to nurse.
- Include human rights and ethical concerns in all discussions about infant-feeding policies.

- Heed the lessons of history, specifically the history of women's almost universal noncompliance with infant feeding guidelines in the past few decades and the history of people's reactions to HIV/AIDS.
- Acknowledge that women inevitably make their own decisions about how they feed their babies. Acknowledge that policy makers in the local area and in international agencies have the power to issue guidelines, but not to enforce "compliance." Acknowledge that they have the power to support (or withhold support from) replacement feeding, but not the power to make women do things that they believe will jeopardize their babies' lives or their own.
- Respect women's ability to reason. Acknowledge that women generally do the best that they can for their babies and themselves.

# References

Appropriate Health Resources and Technologies Action Group. 1997. Caring with Confidence. London: AHRTAG.

Baker, Kristi, and Vivien Nakawala. 1991. Breastfeeding and AIDS survey. *NGO AIDS Newsletter* (Family Health Trust, Lusaka): 2, April 4.

Barbacci, M., J. T. Repke and R. E. Chaisson. 1991. Routine prenatal screening for HIV infection. *Lancet* 337: 709–711.

Barber, Sue. 1998. Infant health best practices: New York. Presented at the Workshop on Infants and AIDS, Sponsored by the Community Nutrition Institute, Washington, D.C., February 11.

Berer, Marge, with Sunanda Ray. 1993. *Women and HIV/AIDS*. London: Pandora Press.

Bertolli, J., et al. 1996. Breastfeeding among HIV-infected women, Los Angeles and Massachusetts, 1988–1993. Presented at the Eleventh International Conference on AIDS, Vancouver, Canada, July 7–12.

Bertolli, Jeanne, et al. 1998. Implementation of recommendations for the medical care of HIV-exposed infants in the first year of life, USA. Presented at the Twelfth World AIDS Conference, Geneva, Switzerland, June 28–July 3. Abstract 23269.

CAFOD. 1998. *CAFOD AIDS Information Exchange Newsletter*, April.

Carusi, Daniela, Lee A. Freeman and Samuel F. Posner. 1998 Human immunodeficiency virus test refusal in pregnancy: A challenge to voluntary testing. *Obstetrics and Gynecology* 91: 540–545.

Coplan, J., et al. 1995. Failure to identify human immunodeficiency virus-seropositive newborns: Epidemiology and enrollment patterns in a white, nonurban setting. *Pediatrics* 96: 1083–1089.

Coreil, Jeannine, et al. 1998. Cultural feasibility studies in preparation for clinical trials to reduce maternal-infant HIV transmission in Haiti. *AIDS Education and Prevention* 10: 46–62.

Goldstein, P. J., and J. Sever. 1996. Preventing perinatal HIV transmission. (Letter.) *Journal of the American Medical Association* 276: 779.

Gostin, Lawrence O., and Zita Lazzarini. 1997. *Human Rights and Public Health in the AIDS Pandemic.* Oxford: Oxford University Press.

Gregson, Simon, Tom Zhuwau, Roy M. Anderson and Stephen K. Chandiwana. 1998. Is there evidence for behavior change in response to AIDS in rural Zimbabwe? *Social Science and Medicine* 46: 321–330.

Greiner, Ted. 1993. Breastfeeding communication strategies, adapted from *Infant and Young Child Nutrition: A Historic Review from a Communication Perspective.* Introduction to *Communication Strategies to Support Infant and Young Child Nutrition,* ed. Peggy Koniz-Booher. Cornell University Monographs 24–25, pp. 7–15.

Ighogboja, I. S., R. S. Olarewaju, C. U. Odumodu and H. O. Okuonghae. 1995. Mothers' attitudes towards donated breastmilk, in Jos, Nigeria. *Journal of Human Lactation* 11: 93–96.

Infant AIDS Treatment Difficult. 1998. *Associated Press,* March 20.

Izazola-Licea, Jose Antonio. 1998. Recommendations from 11 Latinamerica AIDS programs to prevent HIV transmission through breastfeeding. Presented at the Twelfth World AIDS Conference, Geneva, Switzerland, June 28–July 3. Abstract 23323.

Johnson, Saul. 1997. The Pan American Initiative: Report-back. Presented at the Conference on Affordable Options for the Prevention of Mother-to-child Transmission of HIV-1, Johannesburg, South Africa, November 19–20.

Kuhn, Louise, et al. 1997. Child feeding practices and attitudes of HIV-positive mothers. Presented at the Conference on Global Strategies for the Prevention of HIV Transmission from Mothers to Infants, Washington, D.C., September 3–6.

Maher, Vanessa. 1995. *The Anthropology of Breast-Feeding: Natural Law or Social Constraint.* Oxford: Berg.

Mann, Jonathan. 1998. Paralysis in AIDS vaccine development violates ethical principles and human rights. Presentation before Presidential Advisory Council on HIV and AIDS, March.

Mikell, Gwendolyn. 1997. *African Feminism: The Politics of Survival in Sub–Saharan Africa.* Philadelphia: University of Pennsylvania Press.

Nduati, Ruth. 1998. *HIV and Infant Feeding: A Review of HIV Transmission Through Breastfeeding.* UNICEF/UNAIDS/WHO.

New Jersey Department of Health WIC Services. 1995. *Policy and Procedure Manual.* Number 2.18.

*New York State Department of Health Policy on Breastfeeding and HIV.* 1991. Albany, New York: New York State Division of Nutrition.

Payne, Cynthia. 1997. *A radical suggestion for WIC clinics.* Available from lactnet@library.ummed.edu; INTERNET, October 3.

Rotundo, Florence. 1998. Infant health best practices: New Jersey. Presented at the Workshop on Infants and AIDS, Sponsored by the Community Nutrition Institute, Washington, D.C., February 11.

Saadeh, Randa J., Miriam H. Labbok, Kristin A. Cooney and Peggy Koniz-Booher,

eds. 1993. *Breast-feeding: The Technical Basis for Action*. Geneva, Switzerland: World Health Organization.

Saba, Joseph. 1997. Consultation on Infants and AIDS, Community Nutrition Institute, Washington, D.C., July 17.

Savage-King, Felicity. 1998. Breastfeeding programmes and HIV questions. In *Mother-to-Child HIV Transmission: Infant Feeding*, Proceedings of the Twelfth World AIDS Conference, Geneva, Switzerland, June 30.

Tess, B. H., L. C. Rodrigues, M.-L. Newell and D. T. Dunn. 1997. Risk factors for mother-to-infant transmission of HIV-1 in São Paulo State, Brazil. Presented at the Fourth Conference on Retroviruses and Opportunistic Infections, Washington, D.C., January 22–27. Abstract 308.

Thomas, Patricia. 1998. The quest for an AIDS vaccine. *Harvard AIDS Review*, pp. 11–14. Winter.

UNAIDS Joint United Nations Programme on HIV/AIDS. 1996. HIV and infant feeding: An interim statement. *Weekly Epidemiological Record* 71: 289–291.

UNICEF. 1998. *New HIV/AIDS Treatment Will Save Thousands of Children*. New York: UNICEF, March 26.

UNICEF,UNAIDS and the World Health Organization. 1998a. *HIV and Infant Feeding: Guidelines for Decision-Makers*. Geneva, Switzerland: World Health Organization.

UNICEF, UNAIDS and the World Health Organization. 1998b. *HIV and Infant Feeding: A Guide for Health Care Managers and Supervisors*. Geneva, Switzerland: World Health Organization.

Urban, Mike. 1997. Attitudes and practices of infant feeding in HIV-1 infected women in Soweto. Presented at the Conference on Affordable Options for the Prevention of Mother-to-child Transmission of HIV-1, Johannesburg, South Africa, November 19–20.

Wellstart International Expanded Promotion of Breastfeeding Program. 1994. *Final Report of Program in Rwanda, March 1992–April 1994*. Washington, D.C.: USAID.

Woods, Dave. 1997. A national dried milk formula. Presented at the Conference on Affordable Options for the Prevention of Mother-to-child Transmission of HIV-1, Johannesburg, South Africa, November 19–20.

World Health Organization, UNAIDS and UNICEF. 1998. *Technical Consultation on HIV and Infant Feeding, Geneva, Switzerland, April 20–22*. Conclusions.

# Index

U.S. Public Health Service  44
USAID (United States Agency for International Development)  67–68, 101–102, 105, 138

vaccines  10, 43, 167, 186
vaginal cleansing  42, 49–50
vaginal microbicides  155
Van de Perre, Philippe  21, 25, 26, 27, 51, 133, 134
Van Esterik, Penny  65, 74–75, 119, 131, 155, 167, 175
Victora, Cesar  70–72, 82
Vietnam  165
viral load  20, 51, 171
vitamin A  21, 42, 48–49

Waloch, Marek  44
water, unclean  69, 118, 151
weaning  30, 103, 156, 168
weanling diarrhea  168
Wellstart  68, 103
Western Blot  24, 27
Western Samoa  124–125
wet nurses  20, 103, 136, 156, 163, 164, 169–171
WHO International Code of Marketing of Breastmilk Substitutes  65, 106, 115, 119–122, 124, 125–126, 130, 150, 157, 183, 194

Wiktor, Stefan  51, 150
Williams, Cicely  115–116
Women, Infants and Children Program (WIC)  136, 174, 191
Women Organized to Respond to Life-threatening Diseases (WORLD)  153
women's perceptions  152–153
World Alliance for Breastfeeding Action (WABA)  2, 165
World Bank  138, 164
World Health Assembly (WHA)  119, 125, 129–130, 139
World Health Organization (WHO)  2, 8, 11, 64, 67, 70, 73, 78, 84, 98, 105, 122, 126, 130, 132, 133, 134, 135, 136, 139, 152–153, 164, 165, 166, 168, 182, 186

Yoon, P. W.  71–72

Zaire  14, 19, 20, 69, 97, 100, 148, 150, 169, 183; *see also* Congo, Democratic Republic of
Zambia  19, 26, 33, 44, 75, 134, 136, 137, 164, 183
Ziegler, John  19
Zimbabwe  2, 27, 52–53, 104, 107, 123, 130, 135, 148, 152, 183